QUICK SOMATIC EXERCISES FOR TRAUMA RECOVERY

90+ Techniques to Release Tension and Enhance Mental Health in Just 10 Minutes a Day

By

Jerome Woodworth

Dedication

This book is dedicated to all those who have weathered the storms of trauma, those who carry its unseen scars, and those who bravely continue to heal. To my patients, past, present, and future, whose courage and resilience inspire me every day. To Sarah, who rediscovered her laughter after years of silence. To *David,* who reclaimed his strength after feeling shattered. To *Maria*, who found her voice amidst the storm. And to all those who are still navigating the uncharted waters of recovery, may these pages serve as a lighthouse, guiding you towards a brighter shore.

Know that you are not alone. Healing is possible. With each gentle movement, each mindful breath, each act of self-compassion, you are weaving a tapestry of strength and resilience. May this book empower you to reclaim your body, your mind, and your spirit, and step into a life of greater wholeness, joy, and freedom.

TABLE OF CONTENTS

Introduction

Your Journey to Embodied Healing

Trauma is a pervasive force, touching countless lives in ways both seen and unseen. It leaves its mark not only on our minds, where memories and emotions linger, but also deep within our bodies, where tension and unease can become chronic residents. In the aftermath of trauma, we may find ourselves struggling with anxiety, flashbacks, nightmares, or a persistent sense of unease. Yet, trauma's impact extends far beyond these psychological symptoms, often manifesting as physical pain, digestive problems, sleep disturbances, and a heightened sensitivity to stress.

At the heart of this mind-body connection lies the nervous system, our intricate network of nerves and cells that regulates our responses to the world around us. When faced with overwhelming events, the nervous system can become dysregulated, stuck in a state of fight, flight, or freeze. Even after the danger has passed, our bodies may continue to react as if we are still under threat, leading to a cascade of physical and emotional symptoms. This can leave us feeling trapped in a cycle of fear, anxiety, and exhaustion.

While traditional therapies often focus on processing thoughts and emotions, somatic therapy offers a different approach. It recognizes that trauma is not just a story in our minds but a lived experience held in our bodies. Somatic therapy invites us to tune in to the sensations and messages our bodies hold, offering a pathway to healing that goes beyond words. Through gentle movement, breathwork, mindfulness, and other embodied practices, we can begin to release stored tension, soothe our nervous systems, and reclaim a sense of safety and well-being.

This book is your guide to embodied healing for trauma recovery. It offers a practical toolkit of somatic exercises that can be easily integrated into your daily life. Whether you're struggling with the aftermath of a single traumatic event or the cumulative effects of chronic stress, these practices can help you reconnect with your body, regulate your emotions, and build resilience. The exercises are designed to be accessible and adaptable, regardless of your physical abilities or experience with somatic therapy.

By committing to just 10 minutes of practice each day, you can begin to experience profound shifts in your well-being. You may find yourself sleeping more soundly, experiencing less anxiety, and feeling more connected to your body and emotions. As you cultivate a deeper understanding of your inner landscape, you'll gain valuable tools for navigating life's challenges with greater ease and resilience.

Remember, healing is a journey, not a destination. It takes time, patience, and self-compassion. By embracing embodied healing, you embark on a transformative path toward reclaiming your body, mind, and spirit. This book is here to support you every step of the way, offering practical guidance and encouragement as you discover the innate wisdom and healing power within your own body.

Understanding Trauma's Impact: Beyond The Mind, Into The Body

Trauma is an unwelcome guest, leaving lasting imprints on our lives that extend far beyond the initial event. While we often associate trauma with emotional distress and psychological symptoms, its impact runs much deeper, reaching into the very fabric of our bodies. To truly heal from trauma, we must acknowledge and address this profound mind-body connection.

The Nature of Trauma

Trauma can stem from a wide range of experiences, from single, catastrophic events like accidents, natural disasters, or assaults, to ongoing stressors like childhood abuse, neglect, or living in an unsafe environment. Regardless of the source, trauma overwhelms our capacity to cope, leaving us feeling powerless and vulnerable.

The body's natural response to threat is to activate the fight-or-flight response, a survival mechanism that prepares us to either confront danger or flee from it. However, in cases of overwhelming trauma, we may become immobilized and enter a state of freeze, where the body shuts down to protect itself from further harm.

These survival responses are essential for our immediate safety, but when they become chronically activated due to unresolved trauma, they can wreak havoc on our physical and emotional well-being. The stress hormones released during these responses, such as cortisol and adrenaline, can remain elevated long after the danger has passed, leading to a state of chronic stress and hypervigilance.

The Body as a Storehouse of Trauma

Trauma is not simply a psychological event; it is a physiological one as well. When we experience a traumatic event, our bodies imprint the memory of that experience, storing it in our cells and tissues. This is why, even years later, we may find ourselves reliving the sensations of fear, terror, or helplessness that we felt during the original trauma.

These stored memories can manifest in a variety of physical symptoms, including:

- **Chronic pain:** Trauma can lead to chronic pain conditions like fibromyalgia, irritable bowel syndrome, and tension headaches.
- **Muscle tension:** Our bodies may hold onto tension in the muscles, leading to stiffness, aches, and restricted movement.
- **Digestive problems:** The gut-brain connection is well-established, and trauma can disrupt digestion, leading to issues like constipation, diarrhea, and nausea.
- **Sleep disturbances:** Insomnia, nightmares, and difficulty relaxing are common in individuals who have experienced trauma.
- **Weakened immune system:** Chronic stress from unresolved trauma can suppress the immune system, making us more susceptible to illness.

The Mind-Body Connection

Traditional approaches to trauma recovery often focus primarily on the mind, utilizing talk therapy and cognitive techniques to process and make sense of traumatic experiences. While these methods can be valuable, they may not fully address the physical manifestations of trauma that linger in the body.

Somatic therapy, on the other hand, recognizes the inseparable connection between mind and body. It views the body as a source of wisdom and healing, holding the key to unlocking the trapped energy of trauma. By tuning into the body's sensations and messages, we can begin to release the grip of trauma and restore a sense of balance and well-being.

Somatic Exercises: Your Path to Healing

Somatic exercises offer a gentle and accessible way to access the body's innate wisdom and facilitate healing. Unlike traditional exercise, which often focuses on pushing the body to its limits, somatic exercises emphasize slow, mindful movement, breath awareness, and gentle touch.

These practices can help:

- **Regulate the nervous system:** By activating the parasympathetic nervous system, responsible for rest and relaxation, somatic exercises can counteract the effects of chronic stress and restore a sense of calm.

- **Release stored tension:** Gentle movements and stretches can help release muscle tension and pain, allowing the body to relax and find ease.
- **Increase body awareness:** By paying attention to sensations in the body, we can develop a deeper understanding of our needs and emotions, leading to greater self-awareness and self-regulation.
- **Enhance emotional processing:** Somatic exercises can create a safe space for emotions to arise and be processed in a healthy way.

The beauty of somatic exercises is that they can be practiced anywhere, anytime, and require no special equipment. Even a few minutes of mindful breathing or gentle movement can have a profound impact on our well-being. By incorporating these practices into your daily routine, you can begin to cultivate a deeper connection to your body, unlock its innate healing potential, and move toward a life of greater resilience and well-being.

The Science Behind Somatic Therapy: How It Works For Trauma

The human body is a complex and interconnected system, where mind and body are not separate entities but rather intertwined aspects of our being. Trauma, whether a single life-altering event or a series of ongoing stressors, can disrupt this delicate balance, leaving lasting imprints on both our psychological and physiological states. Somatic therapy, a holistic approach to healing, delves into this mind-body connection, offering a scientifically-grounded pathway to recovery from trauma's lingering effects.

The Nervous System: Our Body's Alarm System

At the core of somatic therapy lies the understanding of the nervous system, a vast network of nerves and cells that controls our bodily functions and responses to the world around us. This intricate system is divided into two main branches: the sympathetic nervous system (SNS), responsible for the "fight-or-flight" response, and the parasympathetic nervous system (PNS), which governs the "rest-and-digest" functions.

In the face of trauma, the SNS becomes activated, triggering a cascade of physiological changes designed to help us survive the perceived threat. Our heart rate and breathing quicken, muscles tense, and stress hormones like cortisol and adrenaline flood our system. While this response is essential for immediate survival, when trauma remains unresolved, the SNS can become chronically activated, leading to a state of hyper-arousal and dysregulation.

This chronic stress response can manifest in a variety of physical and emotional symptoms, including anxiety, panic attacks, insomnia, digestive problems, chronic pain, and a weakened immune system. In essence, our bodies become trapped in a state of perpetual alert, even when there is no immediate danger present.

Somatic Therapy: Rewiring the Nervous System

Somatic therapy works by gently guiding the nervous system back into a state of balance and regulation. Unlike traditional talk therapy, which focuses primarily on cognitive processing of traumatic events, somatic therapy engages the body directly, utilizing movement, touch, breathwork, and mindfulness practices to access and release the trapped energy of trauma.

Through these embodied practices, we can begin to soothe the overactive SNS and strengthen the PNS, promoting relaxation, calmness, and a sense of safety. By working with the body's sensations and movement patterns, we can access the deeper layers of trauma that may be stored in our tissues and muscles, allowing for gradual healing and integration.

Neuroplasticity: The Brain's Capacity for Change

One of the most exciting aspects of somatic therapy is its alignment with the emerging field of neuroplasticity, which explores the brain's remarkable ability to reorganize and form new neural connections throughout life. Research has shown that trauma can alter the structure and function of the brain, particularly in regions associated with memory, emotion regulation, and the stress response.

Somatic therapy, by engaging the body and its sensations, can help to rewire these neural pathways and create new, healthier patterns. For example, gentle movement and touch can stimulate the release of oxytocin, a hormone associated with bonding, trust, and social connection, which can counteract the isolating effects of trauma.

The Role of Interoception

A key component of somatic therapy is the cultivation of interoception, the ability to sense and interpret the internal signals of our bodies. By paying attention to sensations like heartbeat, breathing, and muscle tension, we can develop a greater awareness of our internal state and learn to regulate our emotions more effectively.

This enhanced interoceptive awareness can be particularly helpful for individuals who have experienced trauma, as they may have become disconnected from their bodies or have difficulty identifying and expressing their emotions. Somatic exercises that focus on breathwork, body scanning, and gentle movement can help to re-establish this connection and foster a greater sense of embodiment.

The 10-Minute Solution: Quick Somatic Exercises for Trauma Recovery

While the science behind somatic therapy may seem complex, the application of its principles can be surprisingly simple and accessible. This book offers a collection of over 90 quick somatic exercises that can be easily integrated into your daily routine. Whether you have 10 minutes to spare during your lunch break, while waiting in line, or before bed, these practices can provide a powerful antidote to the stress and tension that trauma often leaves behind.

By consistently engaging in these exercises, you can:

- Calm your nervous system and reduce hyper-arousal
- Release stored tension and physical pain
- Improve sleep quality
- Increase body awareness and emotional regulation
- Develop a stronger sense of wellbeing and resilience.

Including somatic techniques in your everyday life is an investment in your well-being and longevity. You can start a life-changing path of healing and self-discovery by respecting the wisdom of your body and treating it with the love and care it needs.

Practical Tools For Everyday Resilience: Your 10-Minute Toolkit

In our fast-paced, demanding world, trauma's tendrils can easily weave their way into our lives, leaving us feeling overwhelmed, disconnected, and stuck in survival mode. But what if there was a way to reclaim your sense of well-being, build resilience, and foster healing, all within the space of a short tea break? Enter your 10-minute toolkit: a collection of practical, science-backed somatic exercises designed to help you manage the impacts of trauma, reduce tension, and enhance your mental health, even amidst the busiest of schedules.

The Power of Small, Consistent Steps

One of the most common misconceptions about healing from trauma is that it requires grand gestures or intensive therapy sessions. While professional support can be invaluable, the truth is that small, consistent actions can have a profound impact on our well-being. By dedicating just 10 minutes a day to somatic practices, you can create a ripple effect of positive change that permeates your entire life.

These exercises are not about pushing yourself or achieving perfection; they are about gentle exploration, self-compassion, and honoring your body's innate wisdom. Whether you're a seasoned yogi or new to the world of somatic therapy, these practices are accessible and adaptable to all levels.

Your 10-Minute Arsenal: A Glimpse into the Toolkit

This book is your personal guide to a treasure trove of over 90 somatic exercises, each one carefully selected for its effectiveness in addressing the physical, emotional, and mental impacts of trauma. Let's explore a few examples of what you'll find in your toolkit:

1. Grounding Techniques:

- **5-4-5-3-2-1 Method:** Use your senses to focus on five things you can see, four things you can touch, three things you can hear, two things you can smell, and one thing you can taste while you use your senses to anchor yourself in the present.
- **Mindful Walking:** As you walk, pay attention to the sensations in your feet and legs, the rhythm of your breath, and the sights and sounds around you.

2. Tension-Releasing Exercises:

- **Gentle Shaking:** Stand with your feet shoulder-width apart and gently shake your arms, legs, and torso to release muscular tension.
- **Progressive Muscle Relaxation:** Begin at your toes and work your way up to your head, tensing and relaxing various muscle groups in your body.

3. Breathwork for Calm:

- **Box Breathing:** Breathe in for a count of four, hold for four, exhale for four, and hold for four. Repeat for several cycles.

- **Alternate Nostril Breathing:** Use your thumb and ring finger to alternately close one nostril while inhaling and exhaling through the other.

4. Mindful Movement:

- **Qigong Flow:** Practice slow, flowing movements that combine gentle stretching, breathwork, and visualization.
- **Yoga for Trauma:** Explore specific yoga poses designed to release tension and promote emotional regulation.

5. Self-Compassion Practices:

- **Loving-Kindness Meditation:** Direct well-wishes towards yourself and others, cultivating a sense of compassion and interconnectedness.
- **Self-Soothing Touch:** Gently place your hand on your heart or belly, offering comfort and reassurance.

6. Nature-Based Practices:

- **Mindful Nature Walk:** Immerse yourself in the natural world, paying attention to the sights, sounds, and smells around you.
- **Earthing/Grounding:** Walk barefoot on grass or sand to connect with the earth's energy.

Why 10 Minutes Can Make All the Difference

The beauty of these quick somatic exercises is that they can be easily integrated into your daily routine. Whether you have 10 minutes to spare in the morning before work, during your lunch break, or before bed, you can find moments to connect with your body and nourish your well-being.

Research has shown that even brief periods of mindfulness and somatic practice can have a significant impact on reducing stress, improving mood, and enhancing overall resilience. By making these practices a regular part of your life, you're not just treating symptoms, you're addressing the root causes of trauma and creating lasting change.

Your Personalized Healing Journey

The exercises in this book are merely a starting point. As you explore them, pay attention to how your body responds. What feels most nourishing? What resonates most deeply with you? Use this feedback to create a personalized toolkit that supports your unique healing journey.

Remember, there's no right or wrong way to practice somatic exercises. Approach each practice with curiosity, kindness, and a willingness to experiment. Trust your body's wisdom, and let it guide you towards greater well-being.

As you consistently engage in these practices, you'll cultivate a deeper connection with your body, develop greater self-awareness, and tap into your innate capacity for healing and resilience. You'll discover that even in the midst of life's challenges, you have the power to create moments of peace, presence, and well-being – all within the space of 10 minutes.

CHAPTER 1

LAYING THE FOUNDATION: GROUNDING AND ORIENTING

Trauma disrupts our sense of safety, leaving us feeling ungrounded and adrift in a sea of overwhelming emotions. But what if you could reclaim your sense of stability, find your footing in the present moment, and begin to heal from the inside out? The answer lies in the power of grounding and orienting techniques. These simple yet profound practices are your first steps towards embodied healing, offering a lifeline back to the present moment and a renewed sense of connection to your body and the world around you.

In essence, grounding is the practice of anchoring yourself in the here and now, bringing your awareness to the present moment through your senses. It's like dropping an anchor into the sea, providing stability and security amidst turbulent waters. Orienting, on the other hand, is about understanding your place in the world, recognizing your surroundings, and knowing where you are in space and time.

Together, grounding and orienting create a powerful foundation for healing. When we're grounded and oriented, we're less likely to be hijacked by traumatic memories or triggered into a state of fight, flight, or freeze. We can begin to cultivate a sense of safety within our own bodies, allowing us to explore and process difficult emotions with greater ease and resilience.

The Science Behind Grounding

Recent research has shed light on the fascinating mechanisms behind grounding's effectiveness. Studies have shown that direct contact with the Earth, also known as "earthing," can reduce inflammation, improve sleep, and enhance overall well-being. This is due to the transfer of negatively charged electrons from the Earth's surface into our bodies, which helps to neutralize harmful free radicals and promote physiological balance.

But grounding doesn't have to involve direct contact with the Earth. Even simple exercises that focus our attention on the present moment can activate the parasympathetic nervous system, responsible for rest and relaxation. This shift in our nervous system state can reduce stress hormones, lower blood pressure, and promote a sense of calm and well-being.

Practical Grounding Techniques

Let's explore some practical grounding techniques that you can easily incorporate into your daily routine:

1. **The 5-4-3-2-1 Technique:** This simple yet effective exercise engages all five senses to bring you into the present moment. Start by naming:

   - Five things around you that are visible to you
   - Four things you can touch (the texture of your clothing, the chair you're sitting on, etc.).
   - Three things you can hear (birds chirping, the hum of the refrigerator, your own breath).
   - Two things you can smell (soap, coffee, fresh air).
   - One thing you can taste (a mint, a piece of fruit, a sip of water).

2. **Mindful Walking:** As you walk, pay attention to the sensations in your feet as they make contact with the ground. Notice the subtle shifts in pressure, the feeling of the air on your skin, and the sights and sounds around you. If your mind starts to wander, gently bring it back to the sensations of walking.
3. **Body Scan Meditation:** Find a comfortable position, either sitting or lying down. Close your eyes and take a few deep breaths. Then, slowly scan your body from head to toe, noticing any sensations that arise. Don't try to change anything; simply observe and acknowledge what you feel.
4. **Holding an Object:** Choose a small object, such as a smooth stone or a piece of jewelry. Hold it in your hand and focus on its texture, temperature, and weight. Notice any sensations that arise as you hold it.
5. **Deep Breathing:** Locate a peaceful area where you can lie down or sit. Grasp your abdomen with one hand and your chest with the other. Feel your tummy rise as you take a slow, deep breath through your nose. Feel your tummy drop as you gently release the breath through your mouth. Continue for multiple iterations.

Modifications for Different Abilities

Recall that these are but a few of methods for anchoring yourself. Try different things to see what suits you the best. If your range of motion is restricted, you can adapt these exercises by just listening to sounds in your environment or by concentrating on sensations in your face or hands.

Whatever method you decide on, the most important thing is to be totally in the present and ground yourself in the here and now by employing your senses. You can develop a stronger feeling of composure, stability, and resilience in the face of life's obstacles by engaging in frequent grounding activities.

Finding Your Footing: Grounding Techniques For Stability And Presence

Trauma can leave us feeling untethered, adrift in a sea of overwhelming sensations and emotions. Our minds race, our bodies tense, and the present moment slips away, replaced by intrusive memories or anxieties about the future. Grounding techniques offer a lifeline back to the here and now, providing a sense of stability and presence that can be profoundly healing.

The Essence of Grounding

Imagine your body as a tree. When a storm rages, the tree's roots anchor it to the earth, preventing it from being uprooted. Grounding exercises function in a similar way, providing a sturdy foundation for your mind and body amidst life's turbulence. By engaging your senses and connecting with the physical world, you can shift your focus away from distressing thoughts and feelings, and into the safety and stability of the present moment.

This shift has a profound impact on your nervous system. By activating the parasympathetic nervous system, responsible for rest and relaxation, grounding techniques can counteract the hyperarousal triggered by trauma. As you practice grounding, you'll likely notice a decrease in heart rate, a slowing of your breath, and a softening of muscle tension.

Grounding Techniques for Everyday Resilience

Here are several grounding techniques, each offering a unique pathway to stability and presence:

1. **The 5-4-3-2-1 Technique:** This classic exercise is a simple yet powerful way to engage all five senses and bring yourself back to the present moment. Start by noticing:

- 5 things you can see (e.g., the texture of the wall, the leaves on a tree, the pattern on your clothing).
- 4 things you can touch (e.g., the coolness of a glass, the softness of a blanket, the roughness of a rock).
- 3 things you can hear (e.g., birdsong, the hum of the refrigerator, the sound of your own breath).
- 2 things you can smell (e.g., coffee brewing, freshly cut grass, soap).

- 1 thing you can taste (e.g., a piece of chocolate, a sip of water, a mint).

2. **Mindful Walking:** Walking is a very effective grounding technique. Observe how your feet feel as they come into contact with the floor while you walk. Experience the push-off of your toes, the roll of your foot, and the heel strike. Observe how your arms are swinging gently and the rate of your breathing. If your thoughts stray, gently bring them back to the memories of walking.

3. **Body Scan Meditation:** Choose a comfortable posture for yourself, such as sitting or lying down on the floor with your feet up. Shut your eyes and inhale deeply many times. Next, gradually focus on everybody component, working your way up to your head from your toes. Take note of any feelings you experience, such as tingling, pulsing, warmth, or cooling. In case you come across any tense spots, take a deep breath and ask them to relax.

4. **Sensory Exploration:** Pick something from your environment, such a silky stone, a sliver of cloth, or an aromatic flower. Investigate its properties with your senses, taking in its texture, colour, scent, and even the sound it produces when you touch it. This concentrated concentration can help you feel calmer and more anchored in the here and now.

5. **Deep Breathing:** Take some time to concentrate on your breathing. Taking a slow, deep breath through your nose, feel your tummy grow. After a few periods of holding your breath, gently release it through your mouth. Continue for a few cycles, observing how each breath causes your body to relax.

Tailoring Grounding to Your Needs

Recall that these are only a few instances of grounding strategies. Try out different practices and discover what works best for you. Some individuals discover that specific workouts work better in particular circumstances. For instance, mindful walking may not be as beneficial as deep breathing if you are feeling overtaken by anxiety.

You can adapt these exercises to your own needs if you have physical constraints. If you can't walk, for example, you can practise a seated body scan or pay attention to the sensations in your hands and feet. Finding exercises that support you in feeling in tune with your body and in the present moment is crucial.

.

Building a Grounding Practice

Make grounding a regular part of your daily practice to reap the full advantages. Allocate a brief period of time every day to hone your selected methods. Grounding can even be included into routine tasks like doing the dishes, brushing your teeth or standing in queue. It will get simpler to enter a grounded condition when you need it most the more you practise.

One effective strategy for trauma rehabilitation is grounding. You can start to heal from the inside out by establishing stability and grounding yourself in the here and now. Recall that getting well is a marathon, not a sprint. Have patience with yourself and acknowledge each little accomplishment as it comes about.

Breath As Anchor: Harnessing The Power Of Conscious Breathing

Following a traumatic event, we frequently experience shallow, fast, or even held breathing. It's as though the very life force within us is restricted, reflecting the tension we bear on the mental and physical levels. However, ironically, that same breath has the capacity to be our most powerful compass, bringing us back to the here and now and giving us a sense of security and serenity.

The Breath-Body Connection

Our neurological system, a complex network that controls our stress response, is directly connected to our breath. Short, shallow breaths are a common sign of tension and anxiety, which activates the sympathetic nervous system (SNS) and causes the production of stress chemicals including cortisol and adrenaline. The parasympathetic nervous system (PNS), sometimes known as the "rest and digest" system, is activated when we consciously slow down and deepen our breathing. This change in the condition of our neurological system can have a significant effect on our wellbeing by lowering blood pressure and heart rate, stimulating relaxation and a feeling of ease, and reducing stress.

Beyond Survival: Breath as a Healing Tool

Breathing is a vital automatic survival mechanism, but it's also an effective self-regulation and healing technique. For millennia, people have utilised conscious breathing techniques, or pranayama in yoga, to support their mental, emotional, and physical health.

We can establish a connection between our conscious and unconscious minds and bodies when we direct our attention to our breathing. We obtain important insights into our emotions, sensations, and wants by accessing the wisdom of our inner experience. Conscious breathing can become a dependable anchor with consistent practice, enabling us to deal more easily and resiliently with tough emotions and situations

Simple Yet Powerful Breathing Exercises

Let's explore some simple yet powerful breathing exercises that you can easily incorporate into your daily routine:

1. Diaphragmatic Breathing (Belly Breathing):

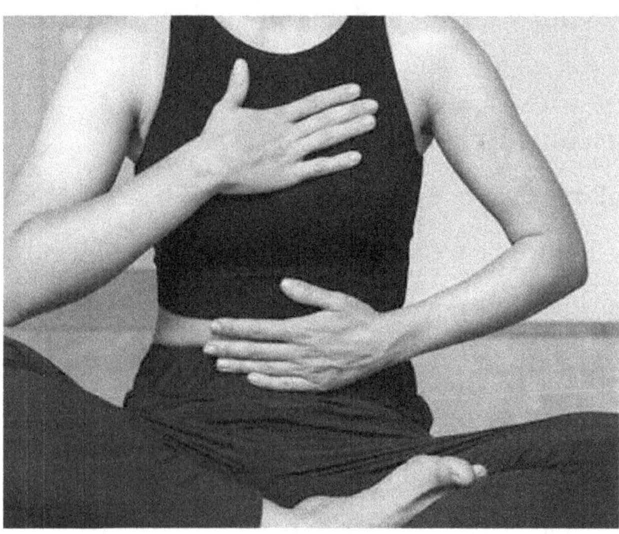

- Maintain a straight spine while lying down or sitting comfortably.
- Hold your tummy with one hand and your chest with the other.
- Breathe in slowly through your nose, allowing your belly to rise as air fills your lungs.
- Feel the fall of your tummy as you gently exhale through your mouth.
- Concentrate on the rise and fall of your tummy as you repeat for five to ten minutes.

2. Box Breathing:

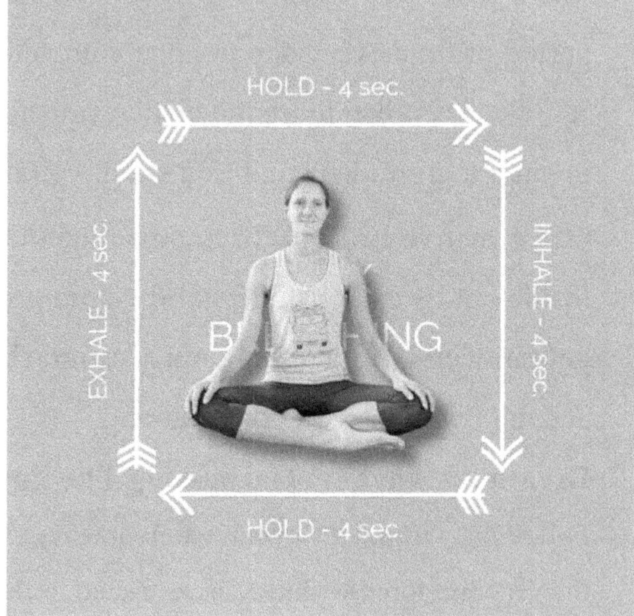

- Take a slow, four-count breath through your nose.
- For four counts, hold your breath.
- Take a leisurely, four-count breath out through your mouth.
- Breathe out slowly and repeat a few times.

3. Alternate Nostril Breathing (Nadi Shodhana):

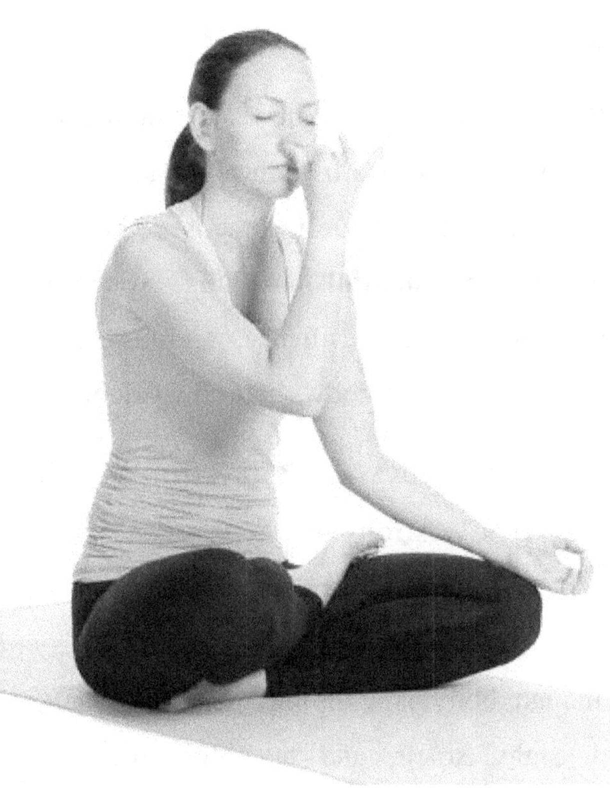

- Sit comfortably, back straight.
- Close your right nostril gently with your thumb.
- Breathe in slowly from your left nostril.
- Release your thumb from your right nostril and use your right ring finger to close your left nostril.
- Gently release the air through your right nostril.

- Take a leisurely breath in through your right nose.
- Shut your left nostril with your ring finger and close your right nose with your thumb.
- Gently release the air through your left nostril.

4. Extended Exhale:

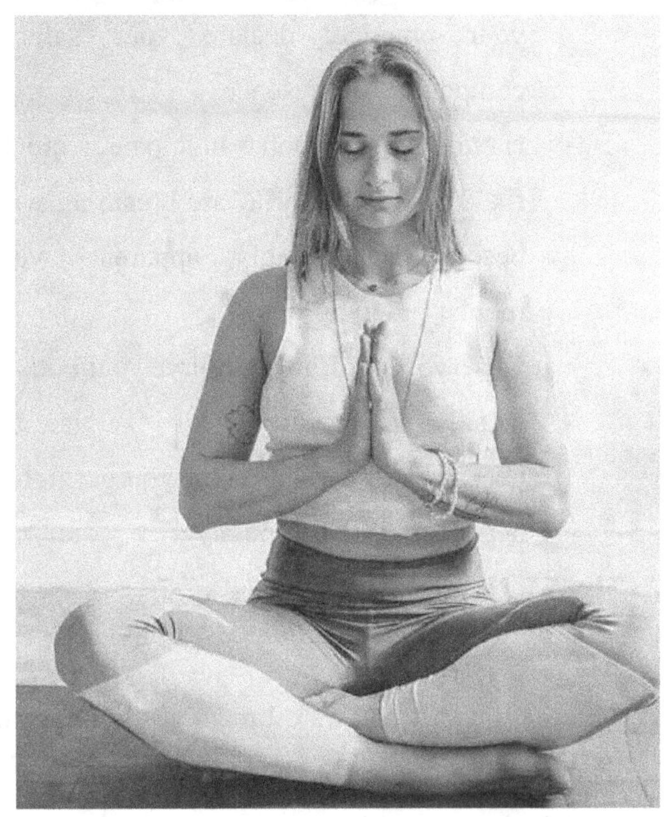

- Breathe in via your nose as usual.
- Gently and completely exhale through your mouth, allowing your exhale to be just a little bit longer than your inhale.
- Continue for a few cycles, extending your exhale with each repetition.

Tips for Enhancing Your Practice

To get the most out of your breathing practice, consider these tips:

- Set up a Sacred Place: Look for a peaceful, comfortable spot where you won't be bothered.
- Establish an Intention: Prior to starting your practice, declare your safety, composure, or presence.
- Have patience: Don't anticipate a quick fix. The benefits of aware breathing will become increasingly apparent with regular practice.
- Observe Your Body: Observe your body's signals and modify your exercise as necessary. Stop and rest if you get light-headedness or dizziness.

Breathing Beyond the Mat

The real benefit of aware breathing is found in incorporating it into your everyday routine, even though these exercises are a fantastic place to

language that speaks to our most fundamental wants, feelings, and experiences. We can revive our body's intrinsic wisdom and set out on a life-

start. Throughout the day, pay attention to your breathing, particularly when you're feeling stressed or anxious. In order to ground yourself in the here and now and trigger your body's natural relaxation reaction, take a few deep breaths.

You'll find that your breath is a continuous companion on your path to healing and self-discovery as you continue to practise. Through the practice of mindful breathing, you can develop inner calm, resilience, and a closer relationship with your body's natural wisdom.

Sensory Awareness: Connecting With Your Body's Wisdom

Sensual Awareness: Harnessing the Wisdom of Your Body

The human body is a living fabric of touch, sound, sight, smell, and taste, an array of experiences. But this music might become muted or altered after trauma. We could lose touch with our bodies, becoming numb to or overwhelmed by the sensations we experience. However, these feelings conceal a deep wisdom—a

changing path of healing and self-discovery by practicing sensory awareness.

Unlocking Your Body's Inner Compass

The practice of purposefully using our senses to tune into the present moment is known as sensory awareness. It involves paying attention to the minute details of both our external and interior landscapes, such as the taste of a ripe strawberry, the sensation of the sun on our skin, and the soft rise and fall of our chest when breathing.

Through developing sensory awareness, we can access the body's innate wisdom, which is a source of knowledge that can direct us towards recovery and wellbeing. Our bodies communicate with us all the time through feelings of ease, warmth, tingling, or tension. These cues frequently provide information about our needs, mental states, and even unresolved traumas.

By developing our ability to recognise these signals, we may start to interpret them and take actions that will further our healing process. To calm our nervous system, we could, for instance, take a few deep breaths, give ourselves encouraging words, or perform a grounding exercise if we feel a constriction in our chest when we recall a previous trauma.

Somatic Exercises for Sensory Awakening

Here are a few easy yet effective exercises that enhance your connection with your body's wisdom and activate your senses:

1. **The Five Senses Check-In**: Stop for a little while and make sure all of your senses are working. Take note:

- **Sight**: What color schemes, designs, and textures are you aware of in your surroundings?
- **Sound**: What sounds do you hear? Are they high-pitched or low-pitched, loud or soft?
- **Smell**: What aromas can you smell? Are they new or old, pleasant or unpleasant?
- **Taste**: Does your mouth still taste anything? Bitter, salty, sour, or sweet?
- **Touch**: Pay attention to how your body feels as it comes into contact with the chair, the floor, or your clothes.

2. **Mindful Eating:** Select a tiny snack, like a chocolate bar or a sultana. Give it a minute to look at it, smell it, and feel its texture before you eat it. After then, put it in your mouth and gradually taste the flavours. As you chew and swallow it, take note of how it feels. You can create a more attentive eating habit and a greater appreciation for food with this activity.

5. **Sensory Exploration Walk:** 5. Sensory Investigation Walk: Take a stroll while keeping a watchful eye on your surroundings. Take note of the leaves, flowers, and trees' various hues, textures, and

shapes. Take in the sounds of the wind rustling the leaves, the birds singing, and the insects buzzing. Feel the soft petals of a flower or the coarse bark of a tree. Remove your shoes and feel the ground beneath your feet if you feel safe doing so.

6. **Mindful Bathing:** Employ all of your senses into your bath or shower. Take note of the sound of the flowing water, the smell of the soap, and the temperature of the water on your skin. Observe how your hands feel on your body while you wash, and how the water feels as it removes the soap from your body.

7. **Texture Exploration:** Collect a range of items with various textures, like a sandpaper piece, a rough wood piece, a smooth stone, and a soft feather. Shut your eyes and examine each item with your hands, noting the minute variations in weight, texture, and temperature.

8. **Beyond the Senses: Cultivating Inner Awareness**

Experiencing the world through your five senses is a great place to start, but sensory awareness goes beyond it. It also entails becoming aware of your inner feelings and experiences. Take note of how your body feels under various circumstances. Do your muscles feel tight or loose? Is your heart relaxed or pounding fast? Do you feel any pressure, warmth, or tingling in your body at all?

You can learn a lot about your emotional condition and your body's requirements by being aware of these internal signs. This knowledge can enable you to make decisions that promote your wellbeing, like taking a break when you're feeling stressed or asking for help when you're feeling alone.

Integrating Sensory Awareness into Daily Life

The beauty of sensory awareness is that it can be practiced anywhere, anytime. Whether you're waiting in line at the grocery store, commuting to work, or enjoying a meal with friends, you can find moments to pause and tune into your senses.

The more you practice, the more natural it will become to be present in your body and aware of the sensations that arise. This increased awareness can help you navigate life's challenges with greater ease, resilience, and joy.

Remember, your body is a wise and compassionate guide. By listening to its messages and honoring its needs, you can unlock a profound source of healing and transformation.

CHAPTER 2

UNWINDING THE PAST: RELEASING TENSION AND TRAUMA

The human body is not merely a vessel for our minds but an intricate archive of our life's journey. Every experience, every emotion, and every trauma leaves a trace within our tissues, muscles, and nervous system. Trauma, in particular, can embed itself deeply, creating knots of tension that linger long after the event itself has passed. To truly heal, we must learn to unravel these knots, releasing the stored energy of trauma and restoring our body's natural flow. Somatic movement offers a powerful pathway to do just that.

The Body as a Barometer

When faced with threat, our bodies instinctively react. Muscles contract, the heart races, and stress hormones surge through our veins. This "fight or flight" response is essential for survival, preparing us to either confront danger or flee from it. However, when trauma goes unresolved, these physiological responses can become stuck, leaving us in a state of chronic tension and hyperarousal.

The body becomes a barometer of our emotional landscape, reflecting the unresolved trauma that resides within us. We may experience tightness in our chest, a knot in our stomach, or a persistent ache in our shoulders. These sensations are not merely physical ailments but messengers from our bodies, urging us to pay attention and address the underlying emotional distress.

Somatic movement practices provide a safe and gentle way to access and process these trapped emotions. By engaging in mindful movement, we create space for sensations to arise and be felt fully. This allows us to reconnect with our bodies, listen to their wisdom, and begin to release the grip of trauma.

The Healing Power of Movement

Movement is not just about exercise or physical fitness; it's a fundamental aspect of human expression and well-being. When we move our bodies, we stimulate the flow of energy, releasing stuck emotions and promoting a sense of vitality and aliveness.

Somatic movement practices differ from traditional exercise in that they emphasize slow, intentional movements, deep breathing, and mindful awareness of sensations. The focus is not on achieving a particular goal or pushing the body to its limits but on listening to the body's subtle cues and responding with compassion and curiosity.

Here are a few simple yet powerful somatic movement exercises to help you release tension and trauma from your body:

1. **Gentle Shaking:** Stand with your feet shoulder-width apart and soften your knees. Begin by gently shaking your hands, then gradually move up your arms, shoulders, and torso. Allow your body to shake freely, releasing any tension you may be holding.

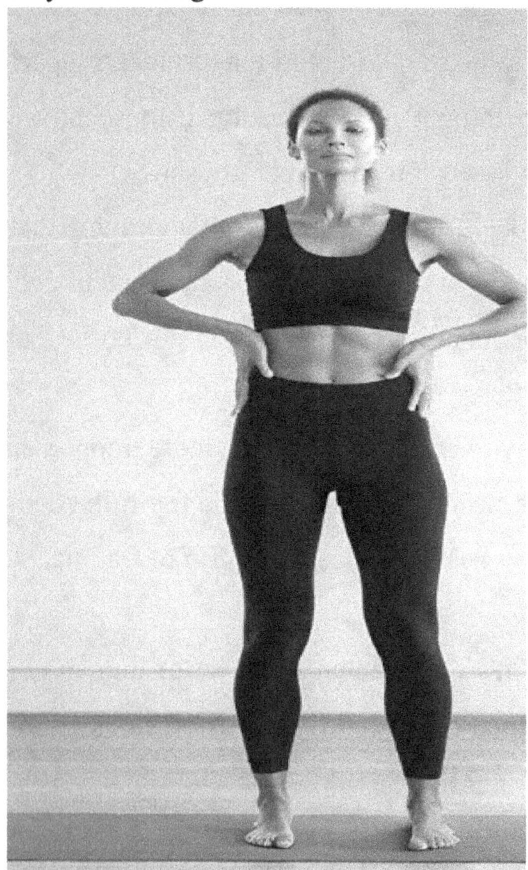

2 **Grounding Sway:** Stand with your feet hip-width apart and gently sway your body from side to side, as if you're a tree swaying in the wind. Feel the weight of your body shifting from one foot to the other, and notice how this movement creates a sense of stability and grounding.

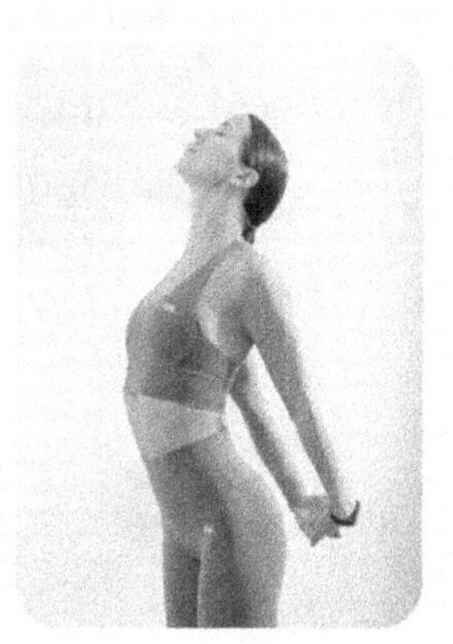
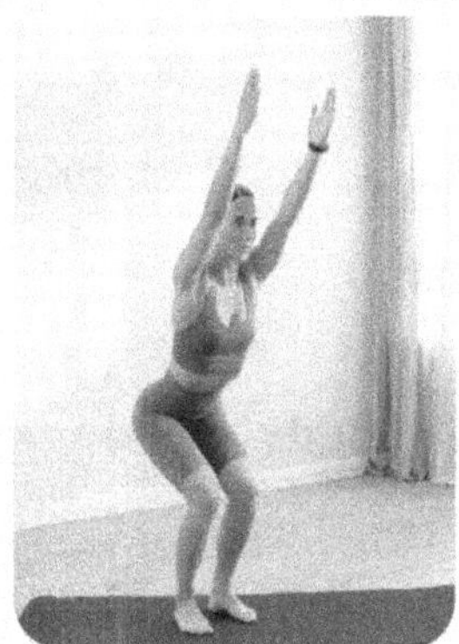

3 Pendulation: This exercise involves alternating between gentle movements of expansion and contraction. Start by reaching your arms overhead and stretching your body upwards. Then, slowly curl your spine downwards, bringing your hands towards your feet. Repeat this sequence several times, focusing on the smooth transition between the two movements.

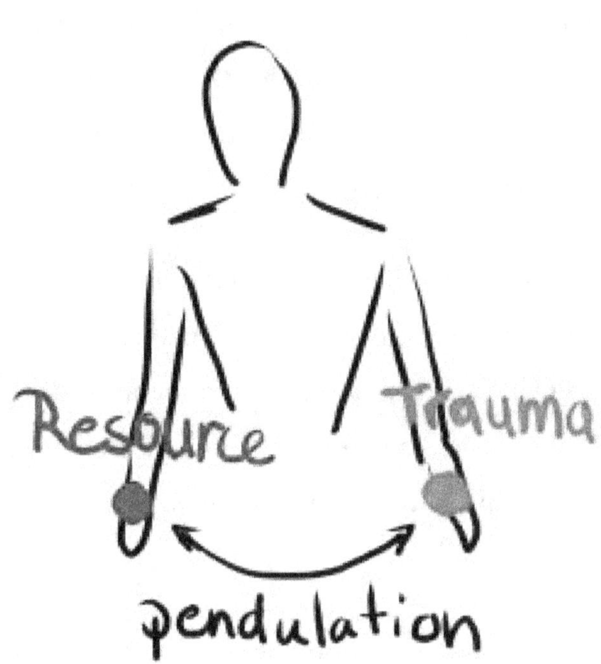

4 Spinal Rolls: Sit or stand with your spine straight. Slowly begin to roll your spine downwards, starting with your head and gradually moving down to your tailbone. Then, slowly reverse the movement, stacking each vertebra on top of the other until you're back in an upright position.

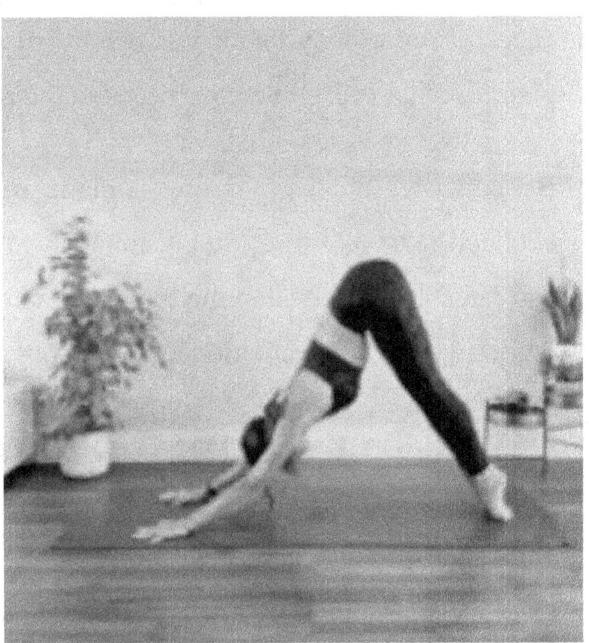

Honoring Your Body's Signals

As you engage in somatic movement practices, it's crucial to listen to your body's signals and honor its limitations. If you feel pain, discomfort, or any other negative sensations, gently adjust the movement or stop altogether. Remember, healing is not about pushing through pain but about creating a safe space for your body to release tension and trauma at its own pace.

Some days, you may feel called to move vigorously, while other days, a gentle sway or a few minutes of deep breathing may be all you need. Trust your body's wisdom and allow it to guide you towards the practices that best serve your needs in the moment.

By consistently incorporating somatic movement into your daily routine, you'll cultivate a deeper connection to your body and its innate healing potential. You'll learn to recognize the early signs of stress and tension, and develop the tools to respond with self-compassion and care. Through movement, you'll unlock a pathway to emotional release, physical relaxation, and a renewed sense of vitality and well-being.

GENTLE RELEASE: SOMATIC MOVEMENT FOR UNBURDENING THE BODY

The profound connection between mind and body is undeniable, especially in the aftermath of trauma. While the mind may strive to compartmentalize and forget, the body holds onto the memory of the experience, often expressing it through tension, pain, and restricted movement. Somatic movement practices offer a gentle, yet powerful way to access and release this stored trauma, allowing the body to unwind and restore its natural flow.

Imagine a tightly wound spring, coiled with the energy of past experiences. Somatic movement acts as a gentle hand, slowly and intentionally unfurling the spring, allowing it to return to its relaxed state. Through mindful movement, we create space for sensations to arise and be felt, fostering a deeper connection to our bodies and the emotions they hold.

Unlike traditional exercise, which often focuses on pushing the body to its limits, somatic movement prioritizes gentle exploration and self-compassion. The emphasis is not on achieving a specific goal or perfecting a pose, but rather on listening to the body's subtle cues and responding with kindness and curiosity.

Let's delve into a few somatic movement practices that can help you gently release tension and unburden your body:

1. **Pendulation:** Begin by standing with your feet shoulder-width apart and your knees slightly bent. Gently rock your weight forward onto your toes, then back onto your heels. Allow your arms to swing naturally as you move. As you continue to rock, gradually increase the range of motion, allowing your body to find its own rhythm. This simple movement can help to loosen tight muscles, improve circulation, and activate the parasympathetic nervous system, promoting relaxation and calmness.

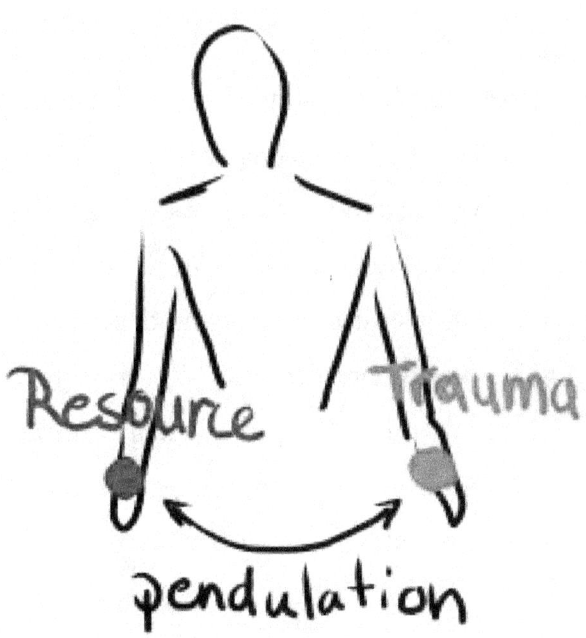

2. **Figure Eight Flow:** Stand with your feet hip-width apart and imagine a figure eight lying on the ground in front of you. Begin tracing the figure eight with your hips, allowing your arms to swing freely in opposition. As you move, notice any areas of tension in your body and invite them to soften. This fluid, rhythmic movement can help to release tension in the hips, lower back, and shoulders, while also promoting a sense of fluidity and ease.

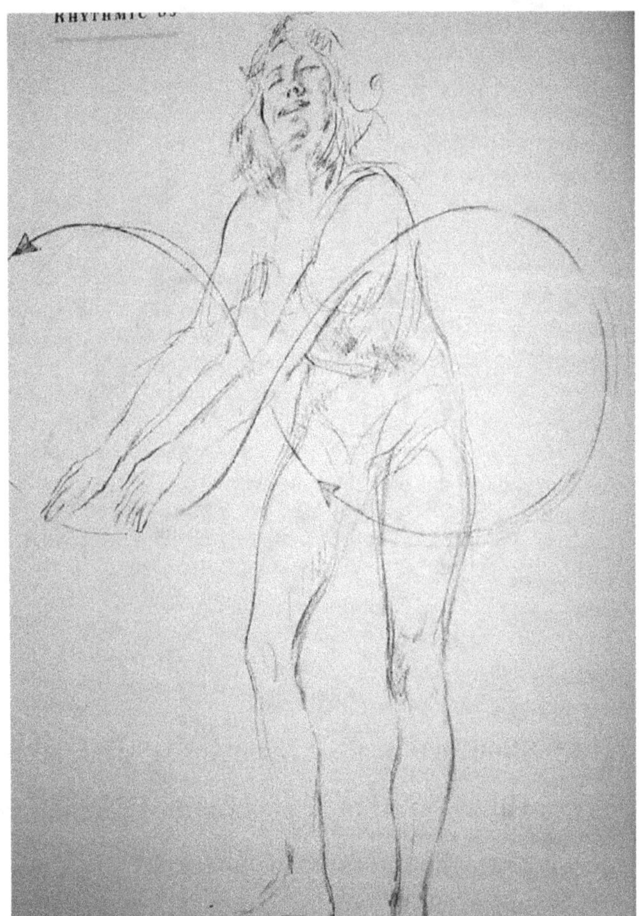

3. **Spinal Waves:** Begin with your hands and knees shoulder-width apart on a tabletop. Taking a deep breath, tuck your chin into your chest and arch your back like a cat. Let out a breath, arch your back like a cow, and lower your abdomen to the floor. Keep moving in this flowing manner, letting the rhythm be dictated by your breath. This mild exercise can aid in increasing flexibility, releasing stress in the neck and back, and mobilising the spine.

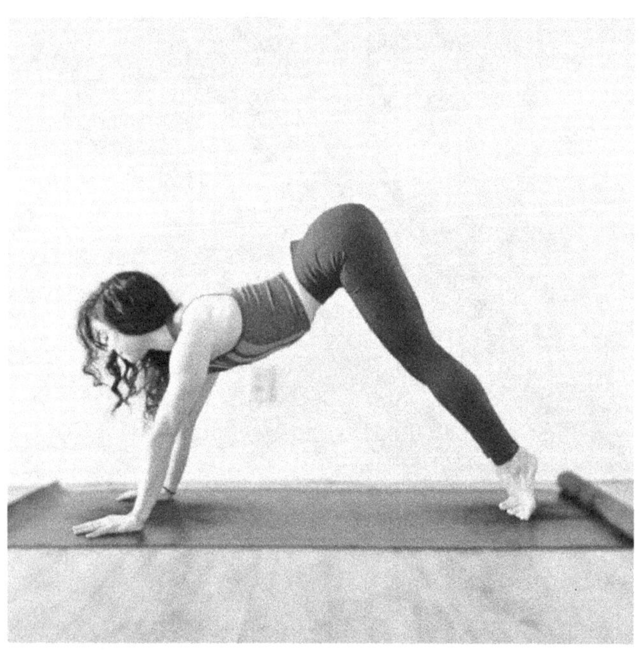

4. **Shoulder Rolls:** Maintain a straight back while you sit or stand. Taking a breath, raise your shoulders to your ears. After a few period of holding, release the air and gently rotate your shoulders back and down. Make numerous repetitions of this motion, paying attention to how smoothly your shoulder blades rotate. By releasing tension in the shoulders and upper back, this exercise can help with pain relief and posture improvement.

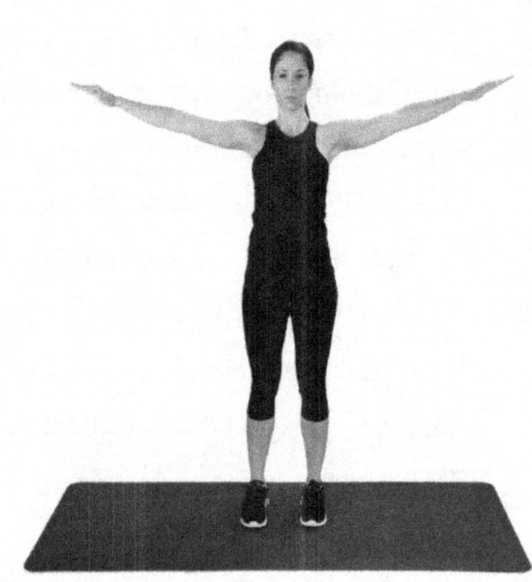

5. **Body Tapping:** Gently tap your fingertips all over your body, starting with your head and moving down to your toes. As you tap, notice any areas of tension and invite them to soften. You can also use your palms or fists to tap, adjusting the pressure to your comfort level. This rhythmic tapping can stimulate circulation, release endorphins, and promote a sense of calm and well-being.

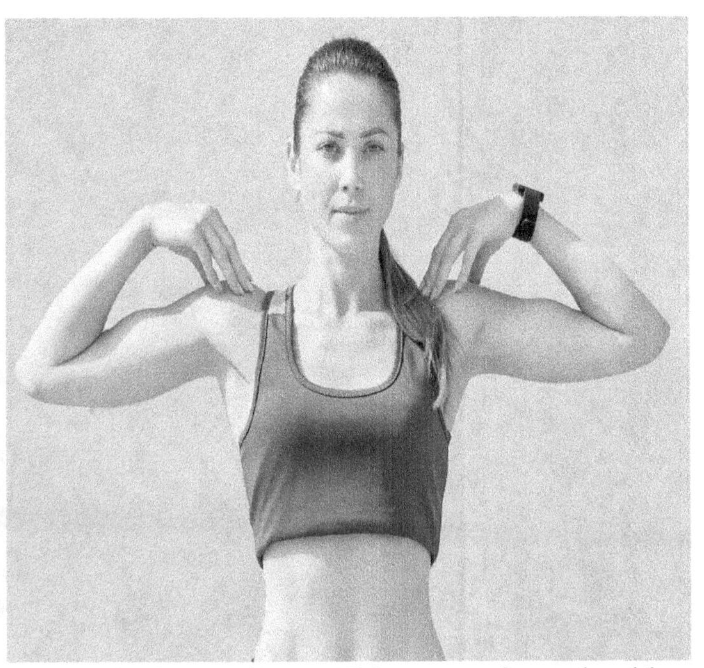 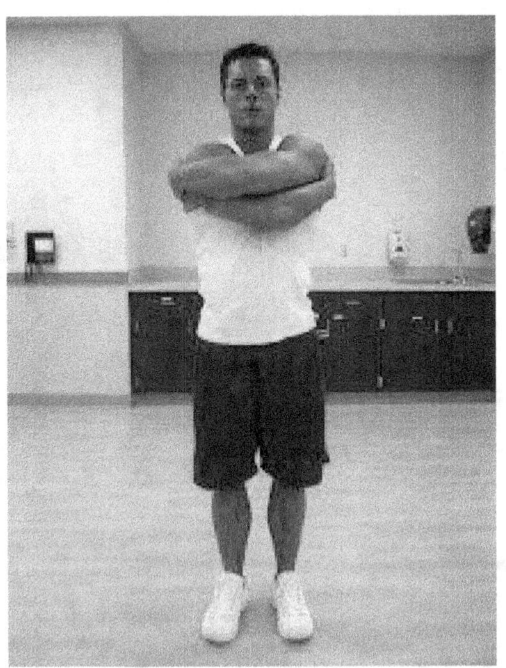

6. **Self-Hugging:** With your feet shoulder-width apart, take a stand and fold your arms across your chest, resting one hand on each shoulder. Give yourselves a warm embrace by loosely putting your arms around one another. Take a few deep breaths, hold, then release and repeat. This small action can trigger the production of oxytocin, also known as the "love hormone," which enhances emotions of security and comfort.

7. **Grounding Through the Feet:** Stand with your feet hip-width apart and your knees slightly bent. Feel the weight of your body sinking into the ground, as if your feet are roots growing into the earth. Imagine the earth's energy rising up through your feet, filling your body with strength and stability. You can also try shifting your weight from one foot to the other, or lifting your heels and toes alternately to further engage your feet and ankles

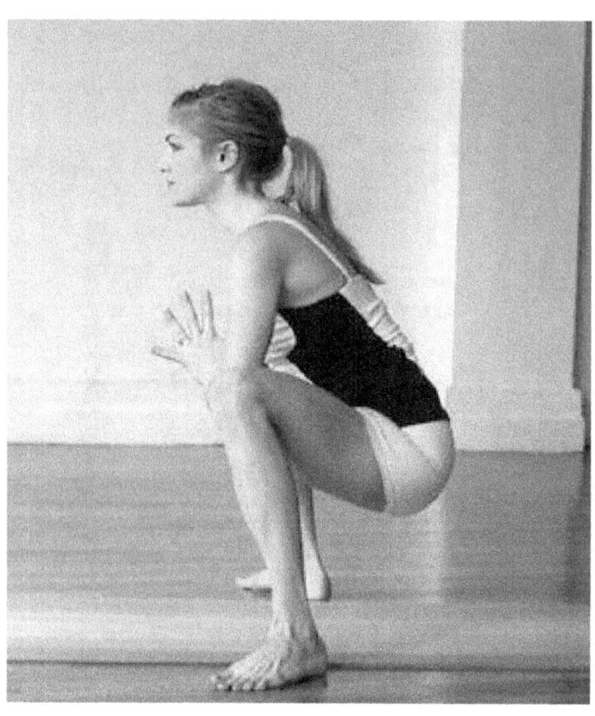

These are just a few examples of the many somatic movement practices available to you. As you explore these exercises, pay close attention to your body's signals. Notice which movements feel nourishing and supportive, and which ones may be too intense or triggering. You should always keep in mind that there is no right or wrong approach move your body The key is to listen to your own inner wisdom and find practices that resonate with you.

By incorporating somatic movement into your daily routine, you'll cultivate a deeper connection to your body and its inherent wisdom. You'll learn to recognize and release tension before it builds up, creating a more spacious and resilient internal landscape. With consistent practice, you'll develop a greater sense of self-awareness, emotional regulation, and overall well-being.

Remember, the journey of healing from trauma is unique for each individual. Be patient with yourself, and trust that your body knows the way. With the support of somatic movement, you can gently unwind the past, release stored tension, and reclaim your body as a sanctuary of peace, vitality, and joy.

Trauma-Sensitive Touch: Self-Care Practices for Emotional Healing

Trauma can fragment our sense of self, leaving us feeling disconnected from our bodies and the world around us. For many survivors, touch can be a trigger, reawakening feelings of vulnerability, fear, or shame. Yet, paradoxically, touch can also be a profound source of healing. When approached with sensitivity and respect, touch can help to restore our sense of safety, reconnect us to our bodies, and foster emotional healing.

Trauma-sensitive touch is not about massage or physical therapy; it's about cultivating a deeper relationship with your own body through gentle, mindful contact. It's about reclaiming your body as a source of comfort and pleasure, rather than a source of pain or fear. By practicing trauma-sensitive touch, you can begin to rewire your nervous system, re-establish trust in your body, and create a safe haven within yourself.

The Science of Healing Touch

Research has shown that touch plays a crucial role in our physical and emotional well-being. When we experience safe, nurturing touch, our bodies release oxytocin, often referred to as the "love hormone." Oxytocin has a calming effect on the nervous system, reducing stress and promoting feelings of connection and trust.

Touch also stimulates the production of endorphins, our body's natural painkillers, which can help to alleviate physical and emotional pain. In addition, touch can activate the vagus nerve, a key component of the parasympathetic nervous system, which plays a vital role in regulating our stress response and promoting relaxation.

Reclaiming Your Body Through Touch

Trauma-sensitive touch is a deeply personal practice, and it's essential to approach it at your own pace and comfort level. Start by simply placing your hands on different parts of your body and noticing the sensations that arise.

You might begin with your hands resting gently on your belly, feeling the rise and fall of your breath. Or you might place your hands on your chest, feeling the steady beat of your heart. As you become more comfortable, you can explore other areas of your body, such as your arms, legs, or face.

Pay attention to the temperature of your skin, the texture of your muscles, and any other sensations that arise. Notice if there are any areas that feel particularly tense or tight, and gently massage or hold those areas with compassion and care.

As you practice trauma-sensitive touch, it's important to honor your body's signals. If a particular touch feels uncomfortable or triggering, stop and try something different. Remember, this is your practice, and you are in control.

Simple Yet Powerful Touch Exercises

Here are a few simple yet powerful touch exercises to incorporate into your self-care routine:

Hand on Heart: Place one hand on your heart and the other on your belly. Close your eyes and take a few deep breaths, feeling the warmth of your hand and the gentle rise and fall of your chest and abdomen.

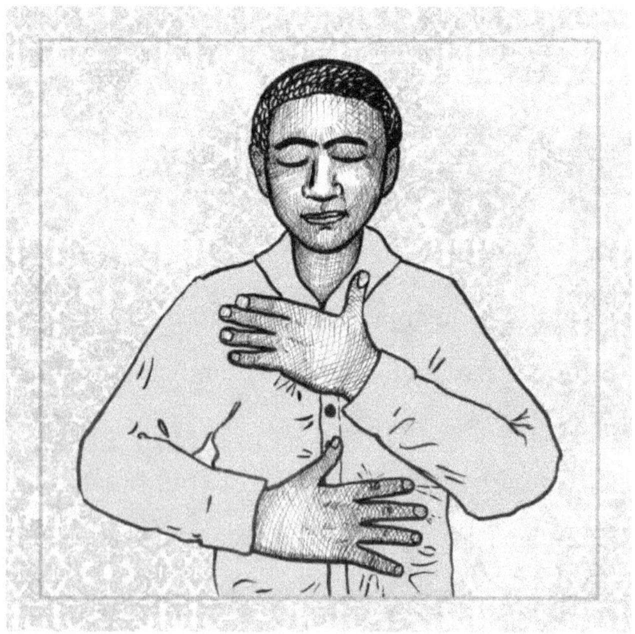

Butterfly Hug: Cross your arms over your chest, placing each hand on the opposite upper arm. Gently tap your fingertips on your arms, alternating sides in a rhythmic pattern. This can help to soothe the nervous system and create a sense of comfort and containment.

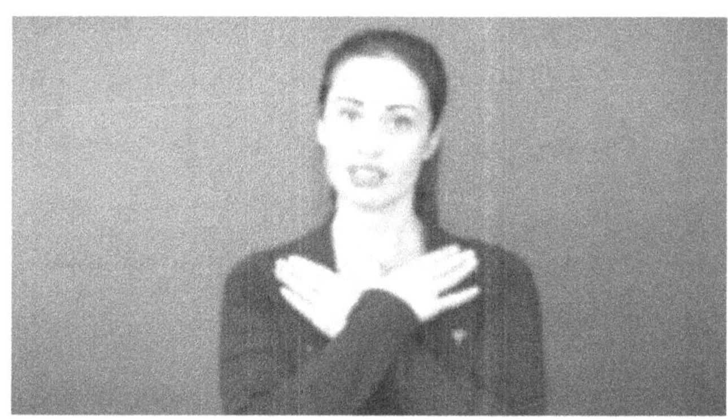

Foot Massage: Sit in a comfortable chair and place one foot on your opposite thigh. Using your thumbs and fingers, gently massage the sole of your foot, working from your toes to your heel. Repeat on the other foot.

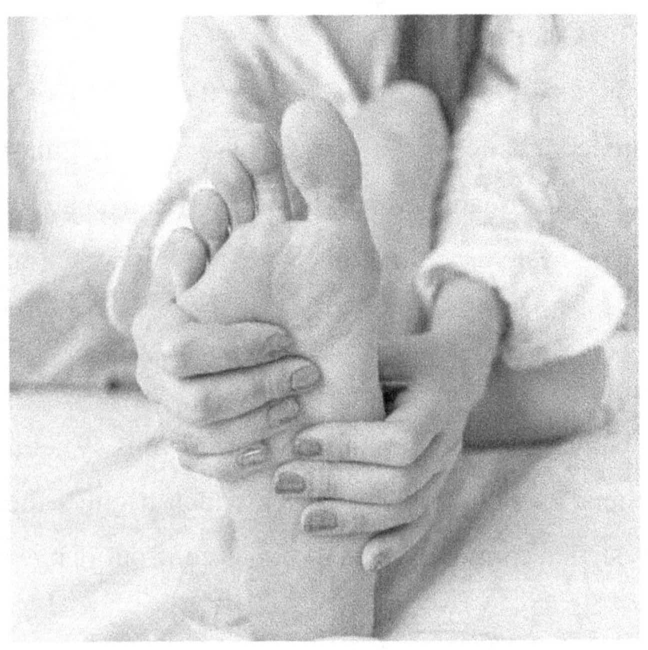

even light tapping. This can aid in relaxing and the relief of tension headaches.

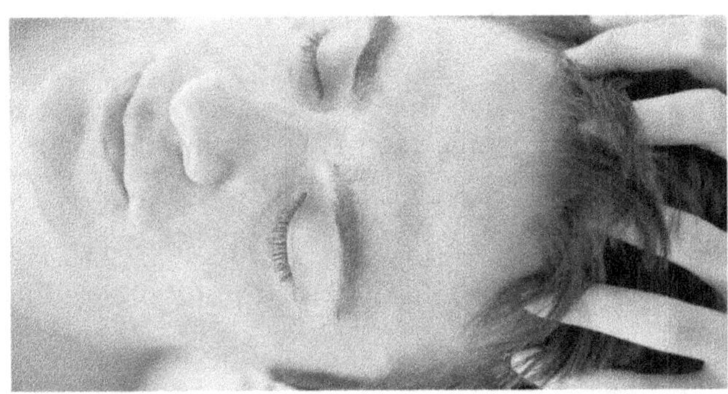

Scalp Massage: Use your fingertips to gently massage your scalp, starting at the base of your skull and moving towards your forehead. You can use circular motions, gentle kneading, or

Holding and Rocking: If you have a partner or trusted friend, ask them to hold you in a gentle embrace. Allow yourself to be held and rocked, feeling the warmth and support of their body. This can be a powerful way to experience safe, nurturing touch and release stored tension.

Creating a Safe Space for Touch

To fully benefit from trauma-sensitive touch, it's essential to create a safe and supportive environment for your practice. Choose a quiet space where you won't be disturbed, and make sure you feel comfortable and relaxed. You can enhance the experience by dimming the lights, playing soothing music, or lighting candles.

Remember, trauma-sensitive touch is not a substitute for professional therapy. If you're struggling with the effects of trauma, it's important to seek support from a qualified therapist who can guide you through the healing process.

By incorporating trauma-sensitive touch into your self-care routine, you can begin to reclaim your body as a source of pleasure, comfort, and healing. With patience, compassion, and mindful awareness, you can transform your relationship with touch and pave the way for lasting recovery and well-being.

Nervous System Regulation: Calming Practices For Overwhelm

The aftermath of trauma can leave our nervous systems in a state of disarray. The world can feel like a minefield of triggers, each one sending us spiraling into anxiety, panic, or shutdown. These overwhelming feelings are not a sign of weakness but a natural response to a dysregulated nervous system. Fortunately, we possess the innate ability to soothe and restore our nervous systems, cultivating a greater sense of calm, resilience, and inner peace.

Understanding the Nervous System's Response to Trauma

To effectively navigate overwhelm, it's essential to understand how trauma impacts our nervous system. When faced with threat, our bodies activate the sympathetic nervous system (SNS), which triggers the fight-or-flight response. This is a survival mechanism designed to mobilize us to either confront danger or flee from it.

However, when trauma remains unresolved, the SNS can become chronically activated, leaving us in a state of hyperarousal. This can manifest as anxiety, racing thoughts, difficulty sleeping, digestive problems, and a heightened sensitivity to stressors. Conversely, some individuals may experience the opposite response—a shutdown or freeze state, where the body becomes numb and immobilized.

Both hyperarousal and shutdown are natural responses to overwhelming experiences, and neither is "better" or "worse" than the other. However, both can significantly impact our quality of life, making it difficult to feel safe, connected, and at ease in our bodies.

Somatic Practices for Nervous System Regulation

Somatic practices offer a powerful antidote to nervous system dysregulation. By engaging the body and its senses, we can directly influence our physiological state, promoting relaxation, calmness, and a sense of safety. Here are a few effective somatic techniques for calming overwhelm:

1. **Orienting and Grounding:**

- **5-4-3-2-1 Technique:** This classic grounding exercise involves noticing five things you can see, four things you can touch, three things you can hear, two things you can smell, and one thing you can taste. This simple practice helps to anchor you in the present moment and shift your focus away from distressing thoughts and feelings.

- **Body Scan Meditation:** Lie down or sit comfortably and systematically bring your attention to different parts of your body, noticing any sensations that arise. This practice can help you to reconnect with your body and cultivate a sense of embodied awareness.

2. **Breathwork:**

- **Diaphragmatic Breathing (Belly Breathing):** by placing one hand on your chest and the other on your abdomen. Feel your tummy rise as you take a slow, deep breath through your nose. Feel your tummy drop as you gently release the breath through your mouth. By stimulating the parasympathetic nervous system, this breathing technique fosters tranquility and relaxation.
- **Extended Exhale:** Inhale normally, then exhale slowly and fully, making your exhale slightly longer than your inhale. This can help to slow down your heart rate and induce a state of relaxation.

3. **Mindful Movement:**

- **Gentle Stretching:** Moderate Stretching: Stretching slowly and gently might help to ease the body and release tension in the muscles. Pay attention to the places on your neck, shoulders, and back where you usually store stress.
- **Yoga for Trauma:** Certain yoga poses, such as child's pose, legs up the wall, and supported savasana, can be particularly helpful for calming the nervous system and promoting relaxation.

4. **Self-Soothing Touch:**

- **Hand on Heart:** Place one hand on your heart and take a few deep breaths, focusing on the warmth and gentle pressure of your hand. This can help to activate the vagus nerve and promote a sense of calm.
- **Butterfly Hug:** Cross your arms over your chest, placing each hand on the opposite upper arm. Gently tap your fingertips on your arms, alternating sides. This rhythmic tapping can have a soothing effect on the nervous system.

Integrating Calming Practices into Daily Life

The key to effectively regulating your nervous system is to make these calming practices a regular part of your daily routine. Even a few minutes of mindful breathing or gentle movement can have a significant impact on your well-being.

- Here are some pointers on how to incorporate these routines into your everyday life:
- **Set Reminders:** Set alarms or reminders on your phone to remind you to take a few minutes for a calming practice throughout the day.
- **Create a Routine:** Establish a daily routine that includes time for self-care and nervous system regulation.
- **Find What Works for You:** Experiment with different practices and find what resonates most with you. There's no one-size-fits-all approach.
- **Be Patient:** It takes time and consistency to rewire your nervous system. Celebrate your accomplishments and have patience with yourself.
- **Seek Support:** If you're struggling with overwhelm or trauma, don't hesitate to seek support from a qualified therapist. They can provide guidance and additional tools for healing and recovery.

By incorporating these calming practices into your life, you can begin to reclaim your sense of peace, balance, and well-being. Keep in mind that you are alone on this journey. With the support of somatic practices, you can learn to navigate life's challenges with greater ease and resilience, and ultimately create a life that feels safe, joyful, and fulfilling.

CHAPTER 3

RECLAIMING YOUR BODY: CULTIVATING AWARENESS AND BOUNDARIES

Trauma can create a chasm between ourselves and our bodies. It can distort our perception of our physical selves, leaving us feeling disconnected, numb, or even ashamed. But within each of us resides an innate wisdom, a deep knowing that can guide us towards healing and wholeness. By cultivating mindful embodiment and establishing healthy boundaries, we can reclaim our bodies as sanctuaries of safety, pleasure, and self-expression.

Mindful embodiment is the practice of paying attention to the sensations, emotions, and experiences that arise within our bodies. It's about being present with ourselves, without judgment or criticism. When we're embodied, we're not just thinking about our bodies; we're inhabiting them fully, experiencing them from the inside out.

This can be a revolutionary shift for trauma survivors, who may have learned to dissociate from their bodies as a means of coping with overwhelming experiences. By reconnecting with our bodies, we can begin to heal the wounds of the past and create a more empowered, integrated sense of self.

The first step towards mindful embodiment is simply noticing. Pause for a short while and become aware of your body. What sensations are you aware of? Is your heart beating fast or slow? Are your muscles tense or relaxed? Are you experiencing any feelings of warmth, coolness, tingling, or pressure?

As you explore these sensations, be curious and non-judgmental. Don't try to change anything; simply observe and acknowledge what you feel. Over time, you'll develop a greater awareness of your body's unique language, which can provide valuable insights into your emotional state and needs.

Here are a few simple practices to cultivate mindful embodiment:

1. **Body Scan Meditation**: Settle into a comfortable position. You can sit or lie down with your feet flat on the ground. Shut your eyes and inhale deeply many times. Next, gradually focus on everybody component, working your way up to your head from your toes. Observe any feelings that surface without passing judgment. Gently return your thoughts back to your body's sensations if they wander, gently bring it back to the sensations in your body.

2. **Mindful Movement**: Select a basic exercise to practise mindfully, such dancing, stretching, or walking. Observe your body's sensations while you move. Take note of your breathing pattern, the feel of your muscles contracting and relaxing, and the contact of your feet with the floor.

3. **Mindful Touch**: Put your hands gently on various body areas, such as your face, chest, and abdomen, to practise mindful touching. Observe your skin's texture and temperature. As you breathe, notice how your chest rises and falls gradually.

Establishing Healthy Boundaries

Another crucial aspect of reclaiming your body is establishing healthy boundaries. Trauma can leave us feeling vulnerable and unsure of our limits. We may have difficulty saying no, setting boundaries with others, or even recognizing when our personal space is being invaded.

By establishing clear boundaries, we create a sense of safety and control in our lives. We learn to say yes to what feels good and nourishing, and no to what feels draining or harmful. This can be a challenging process, especially for those who have experienced trauma, but it's essential for healing and well-being.

Here are a few tips for establishing healthy boundaries:

1. **Listen to Your Body**: Your body is a wise guide. Take note of your feelings in different situations. If you feel uncomfortable, anxious, or overwhelmed, it may be a sign that a boundary needs to be set.

2. Start Small: Setting boundaries doesn't have to be a big, dramatic event. You can start by setting small boundaries with yourself, such as taking a break when you feel overwhelmed or saying no to social engagements that you don't have the energy for.

3. **Communicate Clearly**: When setting boundaries with others, be clear and direct about your needs and limits. Use "I" statements to express how you feel, and avoid apologizing or making excuses.

4. **Practice Self-Compassion**: Setting boundaries can be difficult, especially if you're used to putting others' needs before your own. Be kind to yourself, and remember that it's okay to prioritize your own well-being.

Your Body, Your Sanctuary

By cultivating mindful embodiment and establishing healthy boundaries, you can reclaim your body as a sanctuary of safety, pleasure, and self-expression. You can learn to trust your body's wisdom, honor its needs, and celebrate its unique beauty.

This journey of self-discovery and healing may not always be easy, but it's worth it. By embracing your body as a sacred vessel, you'll unlock a wellspring of resilience, creativity, and joy that will enrich every aspect of your life.

Mindful Embodiment: Tuning In To Your Body's Signals

Trauma can leave us feeling disconnected from our bodies, as if we're inhabiting a shell rather than a living, breathing being. Our senses may become dulled, our emotions muted, and our awareness of physical sensations diminished. Yet, even in the wake of profound pain, the body holds an innate wisdom, a silent language that speaks volumes about our needs, emotions, and experiences. Mindful embodiment is the practice of learning to listen to this language, of reconnecting with our bodies and cultivating a deeper understanding of their messages.

What is Mindful Embodiment?

At its core, mindful embodiment is the practice of paying attention to the present moment without judgment. It's about noticing the subtle shifts in our physical and emotional landscape, the ebb and flow of sensations, and the ever-changing dance between our inner and outer worlds.

Unlike traditional mindfulness practices, which often focus on thoughts and emotions, mindful embodiment emphasizes the body as a primary source of information and wisdom. By tuning into our physical sensations, we can gain valuable insights into our emotional state, our needs, and even our unresolved traumas.

The Benefits of Mindful Embodiment for Trauma Recovery

For those who have experienced trauma, mindful embodiment can be a transformative practice It can help your healing process in the following ways:

1. **Increased Body Awareness:** Trauma often leads to disconnection from the body, but mindful embodiment helps us to reclaim our physical selves. By paying attention to sensations like tension,

tightness, warmth, or coolness, we develop a greater awareness of our bodies and their subtle signals.

2. **Improved Emotional Regulation:** When we're attuned to our bodies, we can more easily identify and manage our emotions. We learn to recognize the physical manifestations of emotions like anger, sadness, or fear, allowing us to respond in healthy and adaptive ways.

3. **Reduced Stress and Anxiety:** Mindful embodiment activates the parasympathetic nervous system, responsible for rest and relaxation. This can help to counteract the effects of chronic stress and promote a sense of calm and well-being.

4. **Enhanced Self-Compassion:** By cultivating a non-judgmental awareness of our bodies and emotions, we can develop greater self-compassion. We learn to accept ourselves as we are, flaws and all, and to treat ourselves with kindness and understanding.

Practical Steps to Cultivate Mindful Embodiment

Here are some simple yet powerful practices to help you cultivate mindful embodiment:

1. **Body Scan Meditation:** Find a comfortable position, either lying down or sitting with your feet on the ground. Shut your eyes and inhale deeply many times.

2. . Then, slowly scan your body from head to toe, noticing any sensations that arise. Don't try to change anything; simply observe and acknowledge what you feel.

3. **Mindful Movement:** Engage in gentle movement practices like yoga, tai chi, or qigong. As you move, pay attention to the sensations in your muscles and joints, the rhythm of your breath, and the way your body interacts with space.

4. **Sensory Awareness Exercises:** Sensory Awareness Activities: Use your senses to learn about your surroundings. Take note of your surroundings colors, patterns, and textures. Play some music or take in the sounds of nature. Use essential oils or aromatherapy to stimulate your sense of smell. Taste food with varying flavors and textures.

5. **Mindful Touch:** Gently place your hands on different parts of your body, noticing the sensations that arise. You can also try self-massage or acupressure to release tension and promote relaxation.

6. **Breath Awareness:** Throughout the day, pause and take a few deep breaths. Notice the rise and fall of your chest and abdomen as you inhale and exhale. This simple practice can help you reconnect with your body and calm your nervous system.

Remember, mindful embodiment is a journey, not a destination. It takes time and patience to develop a deeper connection with your body. Be kind to yourself as you explore these practices, and allow yourself to simply be present with whatever arises.

As you continue to practice, you'll discover that your body is a source of wisdom and guidance. By learning to listen to its signals, you'll gain valuable insights into your emotional state, your needs, and your path to healing. Mindful embodiment empowers you to reclaim your body as a sanctuary of safety, pleasure, and self-expression.

Honouring Your Boundaries: Saying Yes To Safety And Self-Respect

Boundaries are the invisible lines we draw around ourselves, delineating our physical, emotional, and mental space. They are essential for our well-being, yet for many trauma survivors, the concept of boundaries can feel foreign or even threatening. After experiencing a violation of trust and safety, it's not uncommon to struggle with setting limits, saying no, or even recognizing when our needs are being ignored or dismissed.

The Importance of Boundaries in Healing

Boundaries are not walls that shut others out; rather, they are bridges that foster healthy connections. They allow us to define our own needs and preferences, communicate them effectively, and create space for mutual respect and understanding. When we honor our boundaries, we are essentially saying yes to our own well-being, safety, and self-respect.

For individuals navigating the complexities of trauma recovery, boundaries become even more crucial. They serve as a protective shield, preventing further harm and creating a sense of agency and control. By establishing and maintaining healthy boundaries, we can begin to rebuild trust in ourselves and others, fostering a greater sense of safety and security in our relationships.

Learning to Say No

One of the most fundamental aspects of boundary setting is learning to say no. For many of us, saying no can trigger feelings of guilt, shame, or fear of disappointing others. However, it's important to remember that saying no is not selfish; it's a necessary act of self-preservation.

When we say no to something that doesn't align with our values or needs, we're honoring our own integrity and well-being. We're creating space for the things that truly matter to us, whether it's spending time with loved ones, pursuing our passions, or simply resting and recharging.

Here are a few tips for saying no with grace and confidence:

- Be clear and direct: Avoid vague language or excuses. Simply state your no clearly and concisely.
- Offer an alternative: If possible, suggest an alternative that works better for you.
- Don't apologize: You don't owe anyone an explanation for saying no.
- Stand your ground: Don't let others pressure you into changing your mind.

Honoring Your Personal Space

Another key aspect of boundary setting is honoring your personal space. This includes both your physical and emotional space. Your body is your sacred temple, and it's essential to protect it from unwanted touch, invasion, or harm.

Here are some practical steps to help you honor your personal space:

- **Pay attention to your body's signals:** Notice how your body feels in different situations. If you feel uncomfortable, tense, or anxious, it may be a sign that your personal space is being invaded.
- **Set clear boundaries:** Let others know what you're comfortable with and what you're not. For example, you might tell someone that you prefer not to be hugged or touched without your permission.
- **Speak up when necessary:** If someone violates your boundaries, don't be afraid to speak up and assert yourself. You have the right to be treated with respect.
- **Take time for yourself:** It's important to create space in your life for solitude and self-care. This could mean taking a bath, going for a walk in nature, or simply spending time alone in quiet reflection.

Creating a Safe Haven Within

By setting and maintaining healthy boundaries, you can create a safe haven within yourself, a place where you feel protected, nurtured, and empowered. This inner sanctuary can serve as a refuge from the storms of life, a place to recharge and reconnect with your inner strength.

As you continue to practice honoring your boundaries, you'll likely notice a ripple effect of positive change in your relationships and overall well-being. You'll attract people who respect your limits, cultivate deeper connections with those you trust, and experience a greater sense of peace and fulfillment in your life.

Remember, setting boundaries is an ongoing process. It requires courage, self-compassion, and a willingness to prioritize your own needs. But the rewards are immeasurable. By honoring your boundaries, you're not just protecting yourself from harm; you're also opening the door to a life of greater joy, authenticity, and wholeness.

Inner Landscape Mapping: Navigating Sensations And Emotions

Our bodies are intricate landscapes, teeming with sensations, emotions, and memories. Each flutter of the heart, each knot in the stomach, each tingle in the fingertips carries a message, a whisper from our inner world. For those who have experienced trauma, this internal landscape can often feel like a confusing and overwhelming terrain. Yet, by learning to navigate this terrain with curiosity and compassion, we can unlock a profound source of healing and self-discovery.

The Art of Inner Cartography

Inner landscape mapping is the practice of intentionally exploring our internal world, becoming aware of the sensations and emotions that arise within us. It's like creating a map of our inner terrain, identifying the familiar landmarks and uncovering hidden pathways that may have been obscured by trauma.

This process involves more than simply noticing our emotions; it's about connecting with the physical sensations that accompany them. When we feel anxious, where do we feel it in our body? Is it a tightness in our chest, a knot in our stomach, or a tingling in our hands? By paying attention to these bodily cues, we can gain a deeper understanding of our emotional landscape and develop greater capacity for self-regulation.

The Benefits of Inner Landscape Mapping

Inner landscape mapping offers a wealth of benefits for trauma survivors, including:

1. **Increased Self-Awareness:** By exploring our internal landscape, we become more attuned to our emotions and the physical sensations that accompany them. This heightened awareness allows us to respond to our needs more effectively and make choices that support our well-being.

2. **Improved Emotional Regulation:** When we can identify and locate emotions within our bodies, we can more easily manage and process them. We learn to recognize the early warning signs of emotional distress, allowing us to intervene before we become overwhelmed.

3. **Reduced Reactivity:** By understanding our triggers and the bodily sensations that precede them, we can develop strategies for managing our reactions and responding in a more mindful way.

4. **Increased Self-Compassion:** As we explore our inner landscape, we may encounter difficult emotions or memories. By approaching these experiences with curiosity and compassion, we can cultivate a greater sense of self-acceptance and love.

Practical Tools for Mapping Your Inner Terrain

Here are some practical tools to help you embark on your journey of inner landscape mapping:

1. **Body Scan Meditation:** Choose a comfortable position and close your eyes to engage in body scan meditation. From your toes to your head, slowly focus on every area of your body. Take note of any new feelings that you experience, such as pressure, tightness, tingling, warmth, or coolness. Gently return your thoughts back to your body's sensations if they stray.

2. **Emotion Wheel:** An emotion wheel is a visual tool that can help you identify and label your emotions. Start by identifying the primary emotion you're feeling (e.g., anger, sadness, fear). Then, explore the nuances of that emotion, using the wheel to identify more specific feelings (e.g., frustrated, heartbroken, anxious).

3. **Journaling:** Keep a journal to track your emotions and the corresponding physical sensations. Notice any patterns that emerge over time. For example, you might discover that you tend to experience tightness in your chest when you feel anxious, or a knot in your stomach when you feel sad.

4. **Creative Expression:** Use creative outlets like drawing, painting, or writing to express your emotions and explore your inner landscape. Don't worry about creating a masterpiece; simply allow your emotions to flow onto the page or canvas.

5. **Talking to a Therapist:** A therapist can provide guidance and support as you explore your inner landscape. They can help you to identify patterns, develop coping mechanisms, and process difficult emotions in a safe and supportive environment.

Remember, inner landscape mapping is a personal and ongoing journey. There is no right or incorrect method to follow. The most important thing is to approach the process with curiosity, compassion, and a willingness to explore the depths of your being.

By developing a deeper understanding of your inner landscape, you can gain valuable insights into your emotions, needs, and triggers. This awareness can empower you to make choices that support your healing journey and create a life that feels more authentic, joyful, and fulfilling.

CHAPTER 4

MASTERING YOUR EMOTIONS: SKILLS FOR REGULATION AND RESILIENCE

Emotions are the vibrant colors of our inner landscape, shaping our experiences and guiding our interactions with the world. Yet, for those who have experienced trauma, emotions can feel like a turbulent storm, overwhelming and unpredictable. We may find ourselves swept away by waves of anger, sadness, or fear, or trapped in a numbing fog of dissociation.

Learning to navigate this emotional landscape is a critical step in trauma recovery. It's not about suppressing or denying our feelings, but rather about cultivating the skills to recognize, understand, and process them in a healthy way. Somatic practices, particularly breathwork, offer a powerful toolkit for mastering our emotions and building emotional resilience.

The Breath: A Bridge Between Body and Mind

Our breath is a direct reflection of our emotional state. When we're stressed or anxious, our breath tends to become shallow and rapid. Our breathing is deep and slow when we're calm. This intimate connection between our breath and our emotions offers a unique opportunity for self-regulation.

By consciously altering our breathing patterns, we can directly influence our nervous system, shifting it from a state of stress and reactivity to a state of calm and ease. Breathwork activates the parasympathetic nervous system, often referred to as the "rest and digest" system, which helps to slow down our heart rate, lower blood pressure, and reduce the production of stress hormones.

Breathwork as Emotional Alchemy

Think of your breath as a powerful alchemist, capable of transforming raw emotions into a more refined state. When you feel overwhelmed by anger, a few minutes of deep, slow breathing can help to dissipate the intensity, allowing you to respond to the situation with greater clarity and composure. When sadness washes over you, conscious breathing can create a space for the tears to flow, allowing the emotion to move through you rather than stagnate.

Breathwork not only helps to regulate emotions in the moment but also builds emotional resilience over time. With regular practice, you'll develop a greater capacity to tolerate discomfort, navigate challenges, and cultivate a more balanced emotional state.

Breathing Techniques for Emotional Mastery

Here are three powerful breathing techniques to help you master your emotions and cultivate inner peace:

Box Breathing: This simple yet effective technique involves inhaling for a count of four, holding for four, exhaling for four, and holding for four. Repeat for several cycles, visualizing your breath as tracing the sides of a square. Box breathing can help to calm the mind, reduce anxiety, and improve focus.

Alternate Nostril Breathing (Nadi Shodhana): Nadi Shodhana, or Alternate Nostril Breathing, is a balancing breath technique in which you close one nostril while inhaling and exhaling through the other. Using your thumb to close your right nostril, take a slow breath through your left nostril to start. Exhaling via your right nostril, close your left nostril with your right ring finger, and let go of your thumb. Breathe in from your right nostril, shut it, and release the air through your left nose. Continue for multiple iterations. This exercise can lessen stress, enhance mental clarity, and balance your nervous system.

Extended Exhale: This technique focuses on lengthening your exhale, which can have a profoundly calming effect on the nervous system. Inhale normally through your nose, then exhale slowly and fully through your mouth, making your exhale slightly longer than your inhale. Repeat for several cycles, gradually increasing the length of your exhale.

Beyond Breath: Embodied Emotional Expression

While breathwork is a powerful tool for emotional regulation, it's important to remember that emotions are not meant to be suppressed or ignored. They are signals from our bodies, providing valuable information about our needs, desires, and experiences.

Somatic practices encourage us to explore our emotions in a safe and supportive way. This may involve allowing yourself to cry, shake, tremble, or make sounds. It may also involve expressing your emotions through creative outlets like drawing, painting, or journaling.

The key is to create a safe container for your emotions, a space where you feel free to express yourself without judgment or criticism. This might involve setting aside dedicated time for emotional processing, seeking support from a therapist or trusted friend, or simply allowing yourself to be with whatever arises.

Cultivating Self-Compassion

It is crucial that you practise self-compassion as you go out on your emotional exploration trip. This entails being kind and understanding to yourself even while you're having difficulties. Recall that everyone goes through challenging feelings from time to time, and it's acceptable to not feel okay. Giving oneself compassion makes a safe haven for recovery and development. You give yourself permission to be vulnerable and flawed as a human being. Developing a healthy relationship with your emotions and strengthening emotional resilience require this self-compassionate approach.

Breathing For Balance: Techniques For Calming Anxiety And Stress

The human body, in its infinite wisdom, holds an innate key to emotional regulation and stress reduction: the breath. When anxiety or stress takes hold, our breath often becomes rapid, shallow, or erratic. This physiological response is a natural part of our survival mechanism, designed to prepare us for fight or flight. However, when these stressful states become chronic, our breathing patterns can remain dysregulated, further fueling anxiety and tension.

Fortunately, we have the power to re-establish balance and calm through conscious breathing techniques. By intentionally altering our breath, we can communicate directly with our nervous system, shifting it from a state of high alert to one of relaxation and ease. This, in turn, can have a profound impact on our emotional well-being, helping us to manage anxiety, reduce stress, and cultivate inner peace.

The Science Behind Breathwork

The science behind breathwork's efficacy is rooted in the interplay between the respiratory system and the autonomic nervous system (ANS). The ANS is comprised of two branches: the sympathetic nervous system (SNS), responsible for the "fight-or-flight" response, and the parasympathetic nervous system (PNS), which governs the "rest-and-digest" response.

When we're stressed or anxious, the SNS takes over, leading to a cascade of physiological changes, including increased heart rate, rapid breathing, and muscle tension. However, when we engage in slow, deep breathing, we activate the PNS, which counteracts these stress responses. This shift in our nervous system state can lead to a decrease in heart rate, blood pressure, and muscle tension, as well as a reduction in stress hormones like cortisol.

Breathwork Techniques for Calm and Clarity

Let's explore a few simple yet powerful breathing techniques that can help you calm anxiety, reduce stress, and restore balance to your nervous system:

1. **Diaphragmatic Breathing (Belly Breathing):**

• Maintain a straight spine while sitting or lying down.

• Hold your tummy with one hand and your chest with the other.

• Breathe in slowly via your nose, allowing your belly to expand as air fills your lungs. Your chest should not move too much.

• Let your tummy drop as you gently exhale through your mouth.

• Concentrate on the rise and fall of your tummy as you repeat for 5 to 10 minutes.

2. **Box Breathing:**

- Take a slow, four-count breath through your nose.
- For four counts, hold your breath.
- Breathe out slowly through your mouth for four counts.
- Hold your breath for four more counts..

3. **Alternate Nostril Breathing (Nadi Shodhana):**

- Take a comfortable seat with a straight back.
- Close your right nostril gently with your thumb.
- Breathe in slowly from your left nostril.
- Release your thumb from your right nostril and use your right ring finger to close your left nostril.
- Breathe out slowly from your right nostril.
- Gently inhale from your right nostril.
- Shut the left nostril and open the right one.
- Gently release the air through your left nostril.
- Do this five to ten times.

4. **Extended Exhale:**

- Inhale normally through your nose.
- Exhale slowly and fully through your mouth, making your exhale slightly longer than your inhale.
- Repeat for several cycles, gradually lengthening your exhale.

Tips for Maximizing the Benefits of Breathwork

To get the most out of your breathwork practice, consider these tips:

- **Find a peaceful, comfortable place:** Find a place where you won't be bothered and create a calm environment there.
- **Set an intention:** Before you begin, set an intention for your practice, such as "I am calm," "I am safe," or "I am at peace."
- **Be patient and kind to yourself:** Don't get discouraged if your mind wanders or if you find it difficult to focus. Continue practicing by gently returning your focus to your breathing.
- **Practice regularly:** The more you practice, the more easily you'll be able to access a state of calm and relaxation. Even a few minutes of daily breathwork can make a significant difference.
- **Experiment:** Try a variety of breathing exercises to see which one suits you the best.

Integrating Breathwork into Daily Life

Breathwork is not just for moments of acute stress or anxiety. By integrating it into your daily life, you can create a foundation of calm and resilience that helps you navigate challenges with greater ease.

Here are some ways to incorporate breathwork into your routine:

- **Morning ritual:** Morning ritual: Breathe deeply for a few minutes to develop a happy attitude for the day.
- **Before bed:** Wind down with a relaxing breathing exercise to promote restful sleep.
- **During stressful moments:** Take a few deep breaths to pause and center yourself before responding.
- **Throughout the day:** Set reminders to check in with your breath and take a few conscious breaths.

As you cultivate a deeper awareness of your breath, you'll discover its transformative power to soothe your nervous system, calm your mind, and enhance your overall well-being. By embracing breathwork as a regular practice, you can reclaim your inner peace and navigate life's challenges with greater ease and resilience.

Embodied Emotional Expression: Safely Feeling And Processing Emotions

Emotions are the lifeblood of our human experience, coloring our world with vibrancy and depth. They guide our choices, fuel our passions, and forge our connections with others. Yet, for those who have experienced trauma, emotions can feel like a double-edged sword. While they hold the potential for profound healing and connection, they can also trigger overwhelming feelings of fear, shame, or vulnerability.

Unresolved trauma can disrupt our ability to process emotions effectively. We may become stuck in patterns of avoidance, numbing, or reactivity, unable to fully feel and integrate our emotional experiences. This can lead to a host of physical and mental health problems, including anxiety, depression, chronic pain, and relationship difficulties.

Embodied emotional expression offers a pathway to healing. It's a somatic approach that recognizes emotions as not just mental events, but also bodily experiences. When we feel anger, we might notice a clenching in our jaw or a tightening in our chest. Sadness might manifest as a heaviness in our limbs or a lump in our throat. Fear might trigger a racing heart or a churning stomach.

By tuning into these bodily sensations, we can gain valuable insights into our emotional landscape. We can learn to identify and name our emotions, track their intensity, and express them in healthy and adaptive ways.

Creating a Safe Container for Emotional Expression

The first step in embodied emotional expression is creating a safe container for your emotions. This means finding a space where you feel comfortable and supported, free from judgment or criticism. It might be a quiet room in your home, a therapist's office, or even a peaceful spot in nature.

Once you've established a safe container, you can begin to explore your emotions through various somatic practices. Here are a few examples:

1. **Mindful Awareness of Sensations:**

- Start by simply noticing what you're feeling in your body. Are there any areas that seem tight, tense, or uncomfortable? Are you experiencing any sensations like warmth, tingling, or vibration?

- Name these sensations without judgment. For example, you might say to yourself, "I notice a tightness in my chest" or "I feel a warmth in my belly."
- Stay with the sensations for a few moments, allowing yourself to fully experience them.

2. **Movement and Expression:**

- If you feel an impulse to move, allow yourself to do so. This might involve shaking, swaying, dancing, or any other movement that feels natural and expressive.
- Pay attention to how the movement affects your emotions. Does it help to release tension or express intensity? Does it shift your emotional state?
- You can also try vocalizing your emotions through sound, such as humming, sighing, or even yelling (if you have a private space to do so).

3. **Creative Expression:**

- If words feel inadequate, try expressing your emotions through creative outlets like drawing, painting, writing, or music.
- Give your imagination free rein and don't worry about the outcome. The process of creation can be just as healing as the finished product.

4. **Dialogue with the Body:**

- Engage in a dialogue with your body, asking it questions like "What are you feeling right now?" or "What do you need?"
- Listen to your body's responses without judgment. They may come in the form of sensations, images, or even words.
- Trust your body's wisdom and allow it to guide you towards healing.

Cultivating Self-Compassion

Embodied emotional expression can be a challenging process, especially for those who have experienced trauma. It's important to approach this work with patience, kindness, and self-compassion.

The following are some pointers for developing self-compassion:

- Acknowledge your feelings: Allow yourself to feel whatever emotions arise, without judgment or criticism.
- Speak to yourself with kindness: Offer yourself words of comfort and reassurance, just as you would to a friend.
- Practice self-care: Take care of your basic needs, such as eating nutritious foods, getting enough sleep, and engaging in activities that bring you joy.
- Seek support: If you're struggling, don't hesitate to reach out to a therapist or trusted friend.

The Path to Emotional Resilience

Embodied emotional expression is not a quick fix. It's a continuous process of healing and self-discovery. However, by consistently engaging in these practices, you can develop greater emotional resilience, improve your ability to cope with stress, and cultivate a deeper connection to your body and your emotions.

Remember, your emotions are not your enemy. They are valuable messengers that can guide you towards healing and wholeness. By learning to listen to their wisdom, you can transform your relationship with your emotions and create a life that feels more vibrant, authentic, and meaningful.

Self-Compassion In Action: Nurturing Yourself Through Difficult Times

The journey of healing from trauma is not a linear path; it's a winding road with twists, turns, and unexpected challenges. There will be moments of progress and setbacks, moments of clarity and confusion, moments of joy and moments of deep sorrow. In the midst of these emotional ups and downs, self-compassion is your unwavering ally, a gentle hand guiding you through the storm.

What is Self-Compassion?

Self-compassion is not about self-pity or self-indulgence; it's about treating yourself with the same kindness, care, and understanding that you would offer to a dear friend. It's about acknowledging your own suffering, offering yourself warmth and comfort, and recognizing that you are worthy of love and support.

For many trauma survivors, self-compassion can be a radical act. We may have internalized messages of self-blame, shame, or unworthiness, making it difficult to extend kindness to ourselves. Yet, self-compassion is essential for healing. It allows us to be present with our pain without judgment, to soothe ourselves in times of distress, and to cultivate a sense of inner resilience.

The Three Pillars of Self-Compassion

1. **Self-Kindness**: Instead of berating yourself for your mistakes or shortcomings, offer yourself understanding and encouragement. Speak to yourself like you would help someone going through a difficult time.
2. **Common Humanity**: Recognize that suffering is a part of the human experience. You are not alone in your pain. Everyone makes mistakes, encounters obstacles, and suffers setbacks.
3. **Mindfulness**: Observe your thoughts and feelings without judgment. Notice when you're being harsh or critical of yourself, and gently redirect your attention to the present moment.

Cultivating Self-Compassion through Somatic Practices

Somatic practices offer a powerful pathway to cultivating self-compassion. By connecting with our bodies and their sensations, we can develop a deeper understanding of our emotions and needs. This awareness allows us to respond to ourselves with greater kindness and care.

Here are a few somatic exercises that can help you nurture yourself through difficult times:

1. **Self-Soothing Touch:**

- Hold your belly with one hand and your heart with the other. Shut your eyes and inhale deeply many times.
- Notice the warmth of your hands and the gentle rise and fall of your chest and abdomen.
- Offer yourself words of comfort and reassurance, such as "I am here for you," "You are safe," or "This will pass."

2. **Loving-Kindness Meditation:**
- Sit or lie down comfortably. Shut your eyes and inhale deeply many times.
- As you start, focus on loving and caring for yourself. You might repeat phrases like "May I be happy," "May I be healthy," or "May I be at peace."
- Extend these feelings of love and kindness to others, including loved ones, acquaintances, and even those you find difficult.
- Conclude by sending love and kindness to all beings everywhere.

3. **Guided Imagery:**
- Find a quiet place where you won't be disturbed.
- Shut your eyes and visualize being in a peaceful and secure environment. This could be a real place you've been or a fictional place you create in your mind.
- Engage all of your senses as you explore this place. Notice the sights, sounds, smells, and textures around you. Give yourself permission to relax and enjoy the present moment.

Mindful Journaling:
- Spend a few minutes putting your thoughts and feelings on paper.
- Be honest and open with yourself, but avoid self-criticism or judgment.
- As you write, notice any physical sensations that arise.
- Be compassionate and understanding in your response to your feelings.

5. **Gentle Movement:**
- Engage in gentle movement practices like yoga, tai chi, or qigong.
- Focus on the sensations in your body as you move, noticing any areas of tension or tightness.
- Breathe deeply and allow your body to flow with the movement.

Integrating Self-Compassion into Daily Life

Self-compassion is not a one-time event, but an ongoing practice. By incorporating these exercises into your daily routine, you can cultivate a deeper sense of self-love and resilience. Here are a few tips for integrating self-compassion into your life:

- **Notice your self-talk**: Take note of your self-talk: Be mindful of the words you use to express yourself. Are you being kind and supportive, or critical and judgmental?
- **Challenge negative thoughts**: When you notice a negative thought, challenge it with a more positive and realistic one. For example, instead of saying "I'm a failure," you might say "I'm doing the best I can."
- **Practice self-care**: Make time for activities that nourish your body and soul, such as exercise, meditation, spending time in nature, or connecting with loved ones.
- **Seek support:** If you're struggling with self-compassion, don't hesitate to seek support from a therapist or trusted friend.

Self-compassion is an effective technique for recovery as well as growth. By embracing self-kindness, understanding, and mindfulness, you can learn to navigate life's challenges with greater ease and resilience. Remember, you are worthy of love and support, both from yourself and others.

CHAPTER 5

EMBODIED EMPOWERMENT: BUILDING STRENGTH AND CONFIDENCE

The journey of healing from trauma is not solely about releasing the past; it's also about cultivating a vibrant and empowered present. While the previous chapters have focused on grounding, releasing tension, and nurturing emotional awareness, this chapter invites you to step into your strength, vitality, and confidence. Embodied empowerment is about harnessing the power of movement to not only heal but to thrive.

Reclaiming Vitality Through Movement

It's a common misconception that movement after trauma should be gentle and cautious. While it's essential to honor your body's limitations and sensitivities, it's equally important to recognize the transformative power of movement for restoring vitality and energy.

Think of your body as a river. Trauma can create dams that obstruct the flow, causing stagnation and depletion. But through movement, we can begin to dismantle these dams, allowing the life force energy to flow freely once again.

Somatic movement practices, unlike traditional exercise, prioritize mindful awareness and integration. They encourage you to tune in to the sensations in your body, noticing how each movement feels and adjusting accordingly. This mindful approach not only reduces the risk of injury but also deepens your connection to your body and its innate wisdom.

Energizing Movement Practices

Here are a few somatic movement practices that can help you cultivate vitality, strength, and confidence:

1. **Full-Body Shakes:** Stand with your feet hip-width apart and your knees slightly bent. Begin by gently shaking your hands, then gradually move up your arms, shoulders, and torso. Allow your body to shake freely, releasing any tension or stagnant energy you may be holding.

2. **Dancing with Abandon:** Put on your favorite music and let your body move intuitively. Allow yourself to express whatever emotions arise, whether it's joy, anger, sadness, or simply a sense of playfulness. Dancing can be a powerful way to release pent-up energy, boost mood, and reconnect with your body's natural rhythm.

3. **Qigong Flow:** Qigong is an ancient Chinese practice that combines gentle movement, breathwork, and meditation. There are many different styles of qigong, but most involve slow, flowing movements that are designed to cultivate energy, promote circulation, and enhance overall well-being.

4. **Expressive Yoga:** Explore yoga poses that encourage you to express your emotions through movement. For example, you might try Warrior II pose to cultivate a sense of strength and power, or Child's Pose to nurture a feeling of safety and comfort.

The Posture-Emotion Connection

Our posture is not just a reflection of our physical health; it also reflects our emotional state. When we feel confident and empowered, we tend to stand tall with our shoulders back and our head held high. Conversely, when we feel down or defeated, our posture may slump, and our movements may become sluggish.

By consciously adjusting our posture, we can influence our emotional state. Standing tall with an open chest can help to boost confidence and reduce anxiety. Rolling our shoulders back and down can release tension in the neck and shoulders, promoting a sense of relaxation and ease.

Here are a few simple exercises to improve your posture and embodiment:

1. **Mountain Pose:** Stand with your feet hip-width apart and your arms at your sides. Ground your feet into the floor and lengthen your spine, reaching the crown of your head towards the ceiling. Let your arms dangle at your sides naturally while you relax your shoulders.

2. **Shoulder Rolls:** Inhale and lift your shoulders towards your ears. Hold for a moment, then exhale and slowly roll your shoulders back and down. Repeat several times, focusing on the smooth rotation of your shoulder blades.

3. **Chest Opener:** Interlace your fingers behind your back and gently lift your arms away from your body, opening your chest. Take a few breaths to hold, then let go.

Building Inner Strength

While physical strength is important, it's equally essential to cultivate inner strength and resilience. This involves developing the mental and emotional fortitude to navigate life's challenges with grace and courage.

Somatic practices can help to build inner strength by:

- **Increasing body awareness:** When we're attuned to our bodies, we can more easily recognize and respond to stress signals before they escalate.
- **Enhancing emotional regulation:** By learning to manage our emotions through breathwork and movement, we become less reactive and more resilient in the face of adversity.
- **Cultivating self-compassion:** Treating ourselves with kindness and understanding helps us to bounce back from setbacks and challenges.

Remember, the journey of embodied empowerment is ongoing. Be patient with yourself, celebrate your progress, and continue to explore new ways to move, breathe, and connect with your body. By harnessing the power of movement, you can cultivate strength, vitality, and confidence, both inside and out.

Movement As Medicine: Energizing Exercises For Vitality

The human body is not designed for stagnation. It craves movement, rhythm, and the invigorating flow of energy. In the aftermath of trauma, however, our bodies may feel heavy, sluggish, or disconnected. We may retreat into stillness, seeking refuge from the overwhelming sensations and emotions that arise when we try to move.

Yet, paradoxically, movement can be a powerful antidote to the inertia and depletion caused by trauma. Engaging in mindful, intentional movement not only releases physical tension but also awakens a dormant vitality within us. It allows us to reclaim our bodies as sources of strength, joy, and aliveness.

The Science of Movement and Energy

Research has consistently shown the profound impact that movement has on our physical, mental, and emotional well-being. When we move, we increase blood flow, oxygenation, and nutrient delivery to our cells. This not only nourishes our bodies but also stimulates the production of endorphins, our body's natural painkillers and mood boosters.

Furthermore, movement has been shown to reduce levels of cortisol, the stress hormone that can wreak havoc on our health when chronically elevated. This reduction in cortisol not only lowers anxiety and promotes relaxation but also supports a healthier immune system and improved sleep patterns.

Beyond the physiological benefits, movement also has a significant impact on our mental and emotional states. When we move, we engage with the present moment, shifting our focus away from rumination and worry. This can be particularly beneficial for trauma survivors who may be plagued by intrusive thoughts and flashbacks.

Somatic Movement: A Gentle Pathway to Vitality

Somatic movement offers a unique approach to cultivating vitality and energy. Unlike traditional exercise, which often focuses on pushing the body to its limits, somatic movement prioritizes gentle, mindful exploration. It encourages you to listen to your body's signals, honoring its limitations and respecting its wisdom.

The following somatic movement practices are designed to awaken your body's innate energy, revitalize your spirit, and promote a greater sense of well-being:

1. **Full-Body Shakes:**
- Place your feet hip-width apart and bending your knees just a little bit.
- Begin by gently shaking your hands, allowing the movement to flow up your arms and into your shoulders.
- Gradually incorporate your torso, hips, and legs, allowing your entire body to shake freely.
- Experiment with different levels of intensity, from gentle tremors to more vigorous shaking.
- Continue for several minutes, noticing how the shaking affects your energy levels and emotional state.

2. **Dancing with Abandon:**

- Put on your favorite upbeat music and let your body move intuitively.
- Don't worry about choreography or perfection. The goal is to simply move your body and allow the energy to flow freely.
- You can dance alone or with others. Experiment with different styles of music and movement to see what feels most energizing for you.

3. **Qigong Flow:**

- Qigong is an ancient Chinese practice that combines gentle movement, breathwork, and meditation.
- The slow, flowing movements of qigong are designed to cultivate energy, promote circulation, and enhance overall well-being.
- You can find many qigong videos and classes online or in your community.

4. **Expressive Yoga:**

- Explore yoga poses that encourage you to express your emotions through movement.
- For example, you might try Warrior II pose to cultivate a sense of strength and power, or Child's Pose to nurture a feeling of safety and comfort.
- You can also create your own expressive yoga sequence, choosing poses that resonate with your emotions and needs.

5. **Breath-Infused Movement:**

- Combine movement with breathwork to enhance your energy and vitality.
- For example, you might try inhaling as you reach your arms overhead and exhaling as you fold forward.
- Or, you might coordinate your movements with the rhythm of your breath, creating a flowing, dance-like sequence.

Integrating Movement into Daily Life

In addition to these dedicated somatic movement practices, you can also integrate movement into your daily routine to boost your energy and well-being. Here are a few tips:

1. **Micro-Movements Throughout the Day:** Even small movements can make a big difference. Set a timer to remind yourself to get up and stretch every hour, or incorporate simple movements into your daily tasks. For example, while brushing your teeth, do some gentle calf raises or ankle circles. While waiting in line, practice subtle shifts in weight from one foot to the other, or gently roll your shoulders. These micro-movements can help to keep your body from becoming stagnant and promote a sense of aliveness.

2. **Active Transportation:** Whenever possible, choose active modes of transportation over passive ones. Walk or bike to work, take the stairs instead of the elevator, or park your car further away from your destination and walk the rest of the way. These choices not only get your blood flowing and boost your energy but also offer opportunities for mindfulness and connection with your surroundings.

3. **Incorporate Movement into Leisure Activities:** Instead of defaulting to sedentary activities like watching TV or scrolling through social media, choose activities that involve movement. Go for a hike, take a dance class, play a sport, or simply put on some music and dance around your living room. By infusing your leisure time with movement, you'll not only improve your physical health but also enhance your mood and reduce stress.

4. **Find Joyful Movement:** The key to sustainable movement is finding activities that you genuinely enjoy. Experiment with different forms of exercise and movement until you discover what resonates with you. This might be dancing, swimming, hiking, yoga, martial arts, or any other activity that brings you pleasure and a sense of vitality.

5. **Make it Social:** Movement can be even more enjoyable when shared with others. Join a walking group, sign up for a dance class, or find a workout buddy. The social connection and support can enhance your motivation and make exercise a fun and rewarding experience.

The Power of Play

Don't underestimate the power of play! As adults, we often forget how to simply move our bodies for the sheer joy of it. Reclaim your sense of playfulness by engaging in activities that make you laugh, smile, and feel alive. This could be anything from jumping on a trampoline to playing tag with your kids to simply dancing around your kitchen while you cook dinner.

Remember, movement is not a chore; it's a gift. By incorporating mindful movement into your daily life, you'll not only build physical strength and stamina but also cultivate a deeper connection to your body, enhance your emotional well-being, and rediscover the joy of being alive.

Postural Alignment: Embodying Confidence and Resilience

The way we carry ourselves in the world speaks volumes before we utter a single word. Our posture, the alignment of our spine, the set of our shoulders, and the tilt of our head all communicate a silent language of our inner state. For those who have experienced trauma, this language can often be one of defensiveness, collapse, or disconnection. However, through mindful somatic practices, we can rewrite this narrative, transforming our posture into a powerful expression of confidence, resilience, and embodied strength.

The Mirror of the Mind: The Body

The mind and body are not separate entities but rather intertwined aspects of our being. Our thoughts, emotions, and experiences leave their mark on our physical form, shaping our posture and movement patterns. Trauma, in particular, can create deeply ingrained postural habits that reflect the protective mechanisms we've developed to survive.

For example, if you experienced trauma that involved physical or emotional violation, you may unconsciously hunch your shoulders or round your spine as a way to shield yourself from further harm. If you were repeatedly criticized or shamed, you might collapse your chest or avoid eye contact as a way to make yourself smaller and less visible.

These postural patterns may have served a purpose in the past, but they can become problematic when they persist long after the threat has passed. They can lead to chronic pain, muscle tension, and restricted movement. They can also perpetuate feelings of fear, shame, and unworthiness.

By recognizing the connection between posture and emotions, we can begin to use our bodies as a tool for healing and transformation. By consciously adjusting our posture, we can influence our emotional state, shifting from a place of fear and contraction to one of confidence and openness.

Somatic Exercises for Postural Alignment

Here are a few somatic exercises that can help you improve your posture and embody confidence and resilience:

1. **Mountain Pose:**

- Stand with your feet hip-width apart and parallel to each other.
- Distribute your weight evenly between both feet, grounding through the four corners of your feet.
- Gently engage your leg muscles, lifting your kneecaps and firming your thighs.
- Stretch your back and picture yourself being drawn upward from the top of your head by a piece of string.
- Relax your shoulders away from your ears and allow your arms to hang naturally by your sides.
- Take a few deep breaths, feeling your body rooted to the earth and your spine reaching towards the sky.

2. **Shoulder Rolls:**

- Taking a breath, raise your shoulders to your ears.
- Hold for a moment, then exhale and slowly roll your shoulders back and down.
- Repeat several times, focusing on the smooth rotation of your shoulder blades.
- This exercise can help to release tension in the shoulders and upper back, improving posture and relieving pain.

3. **Chest Opener:**
- Interlace your fingers behind your back and gently lift your arms away from your body, opening your chest.
- Maintain your chin horizontal to the floor and your shoulders relaxed.
- Breathe in for a little while, then exhale and repeat.

- This stretch can help to counteract the hunched posture that often accompanies trauma, promoting a sense of confidence and openness.

4. Wall Angels:

- Stand with your back against a wall, feet shoulder-width apart and a few inches away from the wall.
- Bend your elbows and raise your arms to shoulder height, pressing your forearms and the backs of your hands against the wall.
- Keeping your elbows and wrists in touch with the wall, slowly glide your arms up the wall.
- When you reach your maximum range of motion, slowly lower your arms back to starting position.
- Repeat for several repetitions.

5. Cat-Cow Pose:

- With your knees behind your hips and your wrists exactly beneath your shoulders, begin on your hands and knees.
- Inhale and arch your back like a cat, tucking your chin to your chest.
- Exhale and round your spine like a cow, dropping your belly towards the ground and lifting your head.
- Continue this flowing movement, coordinating your breath with the movement of your spine.

Integrating Postural Awareness into Daily Life

In addition to these specific exercises, you can also integrate postural awareness into your daily life. Throughout the day, be mindful of your posture, gait, and seating patterns. Are you slouching at your desk? Are you hunching over your phone? Take regular breaks to stretch and realign your spine.

Here are some additional tips for cultivating good posture:

- Use a supportive chair and adjust it to the proper height.
- When standing, distribute your weight evenly between both feet.
- Avoid crossing your legs or ankles.

- When lifting heavy objects, bend your knees and use your legs, not your back.
- Engage in regular exercise to strengthen your core and back muscles.

By making small adjustments to your posture throughout the day, you can create a ripple effect of positive change in your physical and emotional well-being. You'll not only look more confident, but you'll also feel more grounded, centered, and empowered.

Remember, changing habitual postural patterns takes time and practice. Be patient with yourself, and don't strive for perfection. The goal is not to achieve a rigid, idealized posture, but rather to cultivate a sense of ease, fluidity, and self-awareness in your body.

Strength-Building Practices: Cultivating Inner and Outer Strength

Resilience is not the absence of challenges, but the ability to navigate them with grace, courage, and an underlying sense of strength. While trauma may have shaken your foundation, it's never too late to rebuild, to foster a renewed sense of empowerment both within your body and mind. Strength-building practices offer a pathway to reclaiming your power, fostering resilience, and embracing the full spectrum of your potential.

Strength Beyond Muscle: A Holistic Approach

True strength extends far beyond physical prowess. It encompasses emotional resilience, mental fortitude, and a deep connection to your inner resources. While traditional exercise often focuses on building muscle and endurance, somatic strength-building takes a more holistic approach, recognizing the interconnectedness of mind, body, and spirit.

By engaging in somatic practices, you can cultivate a sense of embodied strength that goes beyond the gym or yoga mat. You'll learn to tap into your inner reserves, harness your innate resilience, and face life's challenges with a renewed sense of agency and confidence.

Physical Strength: Grounding Your Power

Physical strength provides a foundation for overall well-being. It allows us to move through the world with ease, grace, and confidence. For trauma survivors, building physical strength can be a powerful way to reclaim a sense of agency and control over their bodies.

Here are a few somatic exercises that can help you build physical strength:

1. **Bear Crawl:** This primal movement pattern engages multiple muscle groups and helps to build core strength and stability. Start on your hands and knees, then lift your knees slightly off the ground. Crawl forward, alternating your hands and feet, while keeping your back flat and your core engaged.

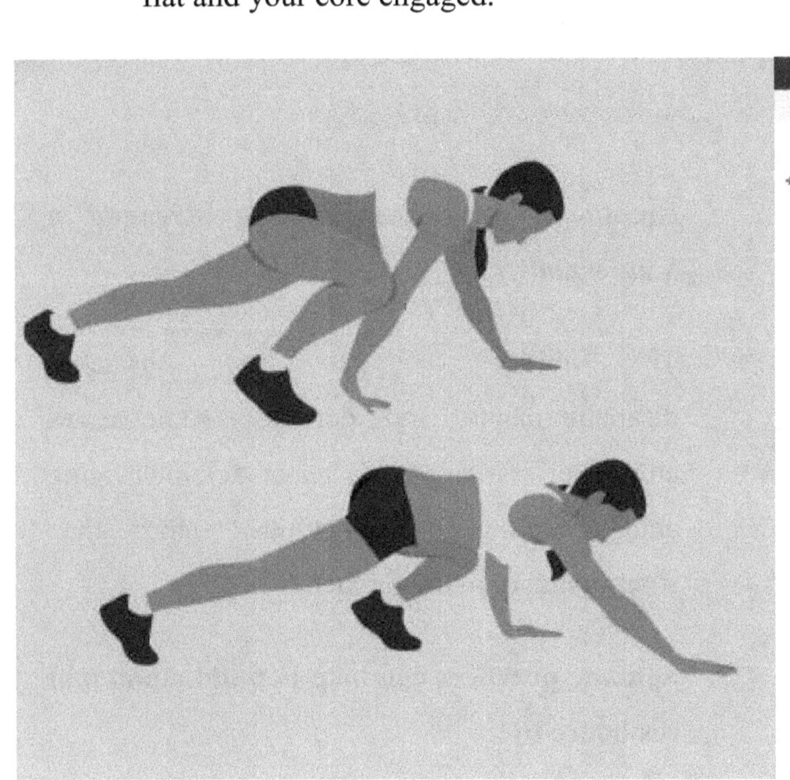

2. **Squats:** Stand with your feet shoulder-width apart and your toes slightly turned out. Bend your knees and lower your hips as if you're sitting back into a chair. Maintain a straight back and an elevated chest. Push through your heels to return to standing. Repeat for 10-15 repetitions.

3. **Lunges:** Stand with your feet hip-width apart. Step forward with one leg and lower your body until your front knee is bent at a 90-degree angle. Maintain a straight back and a contracted core. To stand again, push through your front heel. Repeat on the other side.

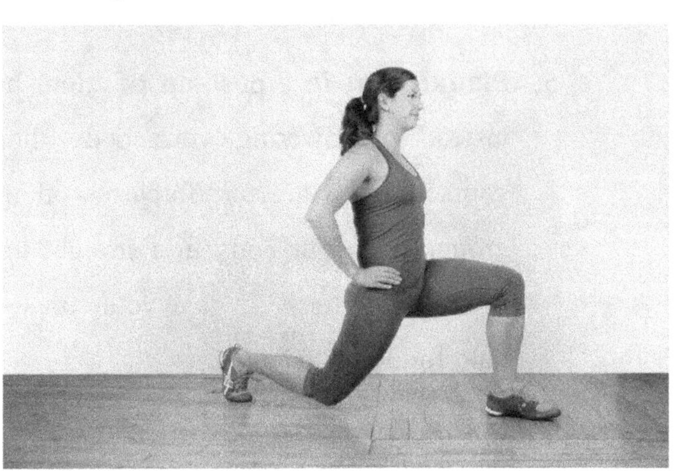

4. **Push-Ups (modified or full):** Start in a plank position, with your hands shoulder-width apart and your body in a straight line from head to heels. Bend your elbows and lower your body until your chest touches the ground. Push back up to starting position. If you're new to push-ups, you can modify the exercise by doing them on your knees or against a wall.

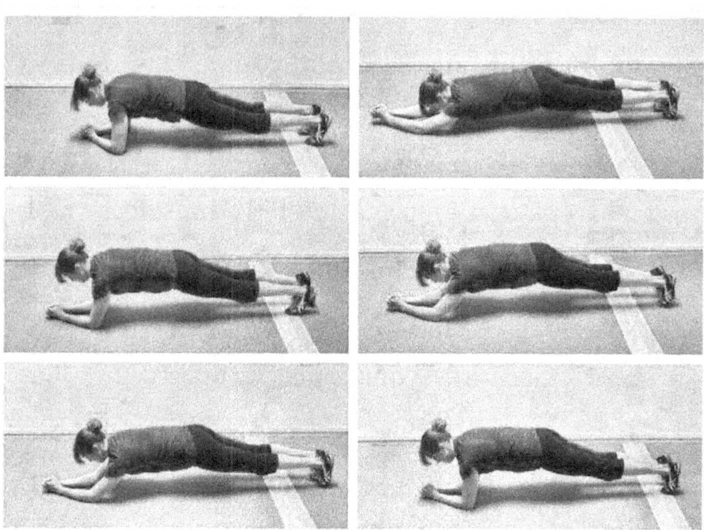

6.

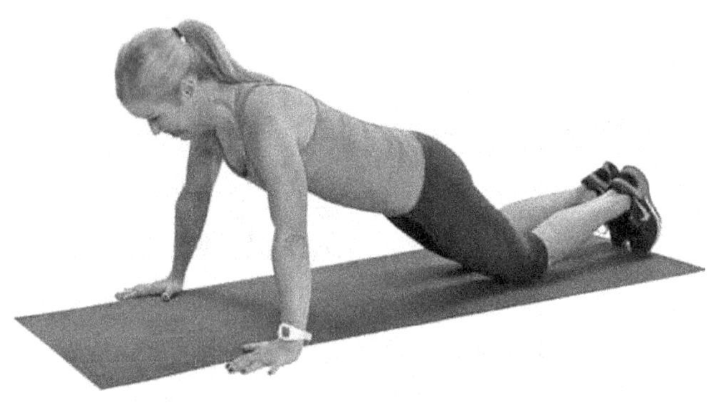

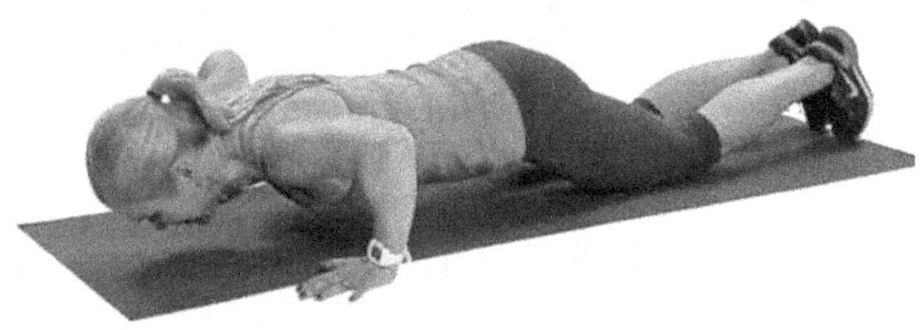

5. **Plank:** Start in a push-up position, but instead of lowering your body, hold yourself up with your forearms on the ground and your body in a straight line from head to heels. Engage your core and hold for 30-60 seconds.

Emotional Resilience: Finding Strength in Vulnerability

The ability to get past obstacles, disappointments, and defeats is known as emotional resilience. It's about acknowledging and accepting our emotions, rather than suppressing or avoiding them.

Somatic practices can help to build emotional resilience by:

1. **Identifying and Processing Emotions:** When you're feeling overwhelmed, take a few moments to pause and tune into your body. Notice where you're feeling the emotion in your body. Is it a

2. tightness in your chest, a knot in your stomach, or a tingling in your hands? Name the emotion and allow yourself to feel it fully.

3. **Self-Compassion:** Offer yourself kindness and understanding, just as you would to a friend who is struggling. Talk to yourself in a gentle and supportive way. Remind yourself that you are not alone and that you have the strength to overcome challenges.

4. **Positive Affirmations:** Create affirmations that resonate with you and repeat them to yourself throughout the day. For example, you might say "I am strong," "I am resilient," or "I am worthy of love and happiness."

Mental Fortitude: Cultivating a Positive Mindset

Mental fortitude is the ability to stay focused, motivated, and determined, even when faced with obstacles or setbacks. It's about cultivating a positive mindset and believing in your ability to succeed.

Somatic practices can help to build mental fortitude by:

1. **Mindfulness Meditation:** In mindfulness meditation, you focus on the current moment while letting go of any judgement. This exercise can help you focus better, lower stress levels, and increase general wellbeing.

2. **Visualization:** Take a few moments to visualize yourself achieving your goals. Imagine yourself feeling strong, confident, and successful. This practice can help to program your mind for success and motivate you to take action.

3. **Goal Setting:** Set realistic goals for yourself and break them down into smaller, achievable steps. Celebrate your successes along the way, and don't be afraid to adjust your goals as needed.

By integrating these strength-building practices into your daily life, you can cultivate a sense of empowerment that radiates from within. You'll develop the physical, emotional, and mental resilience to navigate life's challenges with grace, courage, and unwavering strength. Remember, strength is not about perfection; it's about embracing your imperfections, honoring your journey, and recognizing the boundless potential that resides within you.

CHAPTER 6

TARGETED RELIEF: SOMATIC SOLUTIONS FOR COMMON CHALLENGES

The journey of healing from trauma is not without its hurdles. Sleepless nights, waves of anxiety, and a persistent sense of fatigue can cast shadows on the path to recovery. These challenges, while common, are not insurmountable. By integrating targeted somatic solutions into your daily routine, you can reclaim your rest, soothe your anxious mind, and re-ignite your inner spark.

Sleep Disturbances: A Restless Mind and Body

Insomnia, nightmares, and fragmented sleep often plague those who have experienced trauma. The hyperarousal of the nervous system, a hallmark of post-traumatic stress, can make it difficult to relax and drift off to sleep. Racing thoughts, intrusive memories, and a heightened sense of alertness can keep you tossing and turning long into the night.

Fortunately, somatic practices offer a gentle, non-pharmaceutical approach to improving sleep quality. Trauma-informed sleep hygiene involves creating a calming bedtime routine that signals to your body that it's time to rest. This might include:

- Dimming the lights and reducing screen time in the hour before bed.
- Taking a warm bath or shower.
- Practicing gentle stretches or yoga poses.
- listening to sounds of nature or calming music.
- Reading a book or engaging in another relaxing activity.

In addition to creating a conducive sleep environment, specific somatic exercises can help to calm the nervous system and prepare the body for sleep. Progressive muscle relaxation, where you systematically tense and release different muscle groups, can be particularly effective in reducing physical tension and promoting relaxation.

Breathing exercises, such as diaphragmatic breathing or alternate nostril breathing, can also help to slow down your heart rate, lower blood pressure, and induce a state of calmness.

Anxiety and Panic: Finding Ground in the Storm

Anxiety and panic attacks can feel like tidal waves, washing over you with overwhelming sensations of fear, dread, and physical discomfort. While these experiences can be debilitating, somatic practices offer tools for anchoring yourself in the present moment and riding out the storm.

Grounding techniques, such as the 5-4-3-2-1 exercise, can help to bring your attention back to your senses and away from the spiraling thoughts that fuel anxiety. Focusing on the physical sensations of your body—the feeling of your feet on the ground, the coolness of the air on your skin, the sound of your breath—can create a sense of stability and calm.

Breathwork is another powerful ally in managing anxiety. When panic strikes, our breath tends to become rapid and shallow. By intentionally slowing down and deepening our breath, we can activate the parasympathetic nervous system, counteracting the stress response and promoting relaxation. Box breathing, a simple technique involving inhaling for a count of four, holding for four, exhaling for four, and holding for four, can be particularly effective in reducing anxiety and panic.

Fatigue and Depression: Rekindling Your Inner Spark

Fatigue and depression can feel like heavy weights, dragging us down and sapping our energy and motivation. While these challenges often require professional support, somatic practices can offer valuable tools for rekindling your inner spark and boosting your vitality.

Movement, even in small doses, can be surprisingly effective in combating fatigue and depression. Gentle exercises like yoga, tai chi, or qigong can improve circulation, increase energy levels, and enhance mood. Even a short walk in nature or a few minutes of dancing to your favorite music can have a profound impact on your well-being.

In addition to movement, mindful breathing can also play a crucial role in combating fatigue and depression. Research has shown that deep breathing exercises can increase oxygen flow to the brain, improve mood, and reduce feelings of fatigue.

Cultivating a Sense of Agency

While the specific exercises and techniques offered in this book can be incredibly helpful, it's important to remember that you are the expert on your own body and its needs. As you explore these practices, pay close attention to how they affect you. Notice which ones resonate most deeply with you, which ones bring you the most relief, and which ones may be too triggering or intense.

Don't be afraid to experiment and modify the exercises to suit your individual needs and preferences. The key is to find practices that feel supportive and empowering, that help you to cultivate a greater sense of agency and control over your body and your life.

By incorporating somatic practices into your daily routine, you can gradually build a toolkit of resources to manage the challenges of trauma recovery. There will be successes and failures, obstacles and breakthroughs. But with patience, persistence, and a willingness to listen to your body's wisdom, you can reclaim your rest, soothe your anxiety, and re-ignite your inner spark.

Trauma-Informed Sleep Hygiene: Restorative Practices For Deep Sleep

Sleep, a fundamental pillar of well-being, often eludes those grappling with the aftermath of trauma. The restless nights, plagued by nightmares or insomnia, are not merely an inconvenience but a significant barrier to healing and recovery. Trauma-informed sleep hygiene recognizes the unique challenges faced by trauma survivors and offers a compassionate, holistic approach to reclaiming restorative sleep.

The Impact of Trauma on Sleep

Trauma can disrupt our natural sleep-wake cycle, leaving us in a state of hyperarousal even when we long for rest. The sympathetic nervous system, responsible for our fight-or-flight response, remains on high alert, flooding our bodies with stress hormones that hinder sleep onset and maintenance.

Furthermore, trauma can fragment our sleep architecture, the intricate pattern of different sleep stages that are essential for physical and mental restoration. We may experience more light sleep and less deep sleep, leaving us feeling unrefreshed even after a full night's rest. Nightmares and night terrors, a common symptom of post-traumatic stress disorder (PTSD), can further disrupt sleep, leading to anxiety and fear around bedtime.

Trauma-Informed Sleep Hygiene: A Holistic Approach

Trauma-informed sleep hygiene is not simply about following a set of rules; it's about creating a personalized routine that addresses the unique needs of trauma survivors. This involves cultivating a sense of safety and relaxation before bed, regulating the nervous system, and establishing healthy sleep habits.

Here are some key principles of trauma-informed sleep hygiene:

1. **Prioritize Safety and Comfort:**

- Create a sleep sanctuary: Make your bedroom a haven of tranquility. Ensure it's dark, quiet, and cool, with comfortable bedding and minimal distractions.
- Establish a calming bedtime routine: Engage in relaxing activities before bed, such as taking a warm bath, reading a book, or listening to soothing music.
- Avoid stimulating activities: Limit exposure to screens and caffeine in the hours leading up to bedtime.

2. **Regulate the Nervous System:**

- Practice somatic exercises: Incorporate gentle movement, stretching, or yoga into your evening routine to release tension and calm the nervous system.
- Breathwork for relaxation: Engage in deep breathing exercises like diaphragmatic breathing or alternate nostril breathing to activate the parasympathetic nervous system and promote relaxation.
- Progressive muscle relaxation involves tensing and relaxing various body parts, beginning with your toes and progressing towards your head.

3. **Establish Healthy Sleep Habits:**

- Maintain a regular sleep schedule: To help your body's normal sleep-wake cycle, go to bed and wake up at the same time every day, including on weekends.
- Avoid napping: Napping during the day can interfere with nighttime sleep. If you must nap, only for 20 to 30 minutes at most.
- Limit your intake of alcohol and caffeine since they can both interfere with your sleep. Steer clear of them in the hours before bed.

- Create a relaxing bedtime ritual: Develop a soothing routine that signals to your body that it's time to wind down and prepare for sleep.

Somatic Exercises for Sleep

Here are some specific somatic exercises that can promote relaxation and improve sleep quality:

1. **Body Scan Meditation:**

- find a comfortable place to lie down while Close your eyes
- Slowly bring your attention to each part of your body, starting with your toes and moving up to your head.
- Notice any sensations that arise without judgment. Simply observe and acknowledge them.

2. **Guided Imagery:**

- Close your eyes and choose a comfortable position to begin guided imagery.
- Visualise yourself in a peaceful comfortable place. A beach, a forest, or any other location that makes you feel at ease could be this.
- As you picture yourself in this location, use all of your senses. What senses do you use? Taste, smell, taste, touch?

3. **Yoga Nidra:**

- Yoga Nidra, also known as yogic sleep, is a guided meditation practice that promotes deep relaxation and sleep.
- You can find many Yoga Nidra recordings online or through apps.

4. **Legs Up the Wall Pose:**

- Lie on your back with your buttocks against a wall and your legs extended up the wall.
- Place your arms by your sides, palms facing up.
- Close your eyes and breathe deeply.
- This pose can help to calm the nervous system and reduce stress.

5. **Child's Pose:**

- Sit back on your heels while kneeling on the ground.
- Fold forward, resting your forehead on the ground and your arms by your sides.
- Inhale deeply, then ease into the position.
- This gentle stretch can help to release tension in the back and shoulders and promote relaxation.

Additional Tips for Restful Sleep

- Keep a sleep diary: Track your sleep patterns, noting any factors that seem to affect your sleep quality.
- Avoid clock-watching: If you find yourself lying awake, resist the urge to check the clock. This can increase anxiety and make it harder to fall asleep.
- Get regular exercise: Exercise can improve sleep quality, but avoid vigorous activity too close to bedtime.
- Create a sleep-conducive environment: Make sure your bedroom is dark, quiet, cool, and comfortable.

Remember, improving sleep is a process that takes time and patience. By incorporating trauma-informed sleep hygiene and somatic practices into your routine, you can gradually reclaim restorative sleep, enhance your well-being, and support your journey of healing and recovery.

Navigating Overwhelm: Somatic Tools For Anxiety And Panic

Anxiety and panic, the unwelcome companions of trauma, can strike like lightning, leaving you feeling breathless, disoriented, and trapped in a whirlwind of fear. These intense emotional states can be triggered by seemingly innocuous events, resurrecting the terror of past experiences and hijacking your nervous system. But even in the midst of the storm, you possess an arsenal of somatic tools to help you weather the onslaught and reclaim your equilibrium.

Unmasking the Anxiety-Panic Cycle

Anxiety and panic are not merely emotions; they are physiological experiences rooted in the nervous system's response to perceived threat. When triggered, the sympathetic nervous system floods your body with stress hormones like adrenaline and cortisol, preparing you for fight or flight.

This response can manifest as a racing heart, rapid breathing, trembling, sweating, and a sense of impending doom. The mind races with catastrophic thoughts, further fueling the cycle of fear and panic.

Somatic approaches offer a way to interrupt this cycle, calming the nervous system and restoring a sense of safety and control. By grounding yourself in the present moment, regulating your breath, and engaging in mindful movement, you can create a safe haven within your own body.

Grounding Techniques: Anchoring in the Present

When anxiety or panic strikes, your mind may race with thoughts of the past or future. Grounding techniques help to bring your attention back to the present moment, where you are safe and the threat is no longer present.

1. **The 5-4-3-2-1 Technique: Engage your senses to anchor yourself in the here and now. Notice:**

   - Five things you can see
   - Four things you can touch
   - Three things you can hear
   - Two things you can smell
   - One thing you can taste

This simple exercise can help to shift your focus away from distressing thoughts and ground you in the physical reality of your surroundings.

2. **Sensory Grounding with a Grounding Object:**

   - Choose a small object, such as a smooth stone, a piece of jewelry, or a stress ball.
   - As you hold the thing in your hand, pay attention to its weight, texture, and temperature.
   - Notice any sensations that arise as you hold it.
   - This tactile focus can help to anchor you in the present moment and distract you from anxious thoughts.

Breathwork for Calm and Clarity

Breathing is a powerful tool for regulating the nervous system and reducing anxiety. When we're anxious, our breath tends to be shallow and rapid. By intentionally slowing down and deepening our breath, we can activate the parasympathetic nervous system, promoting relaxation and calmness.

1. **Diaphragmatic Breathing (Belly Breathing):**

- Sit or lie down comfortably with your spine straight.
- Put your hands on your belly and your chest, respectively.
- Take a slow, deep breath through your nose. As your lungs fill with air, feel your belly rise. Your chest should stay mostly motionless.
- Slowly release the air through your mouth, letting your stomach drop.
- Concentrate on the rise and fall of your belly as you repeat this for a few minutes.

2. **Box Breathing:**

- Inhale slowly for a count of four.
- For four counts, hold your breath.
- Breathe out slowly four times.
- Once more, hold your breath for four counts.
- Repeat for several cycles.

3. **Alternate Nostril Breathing (Nadi Shodhana):**

- Use your thumb and ring finger to alternately close one nostril while inhaling and exhaling through the other.
- Inhale through your left nostril, close it, and exhale through your right nostril.
- Then, inhale through your right nostril, close it, and exhale through your left.
- Repeat for several cycles.

Mindful Movement for Emotional Release

Gentle movement can help to release the physical tension that often accompanies anxiety and panic. It can also serve as a distraction from anxious thoughts and help you to reconnect with your body.

1. **Gentle Rocking:**

- Sit in a comfortable chair and gently rock your body back and forth.
- As you move, let your arms swing naturally.

- Focus on the sensations of rocking and the rhythm of your breath.

2. **Progressive Muscle Relaxation:**

- Starting with your toes, tense each muscle group in your body for a few seconds, then release.
- Tensing and relaxing each muscle group as you go up your body, continue until you reach your head.

3. **Simple Stretches:**

- Stand or sit comfortably and gently stretch your arms, neck, and back.
- Hold each stretch for a few breaths, then release.
- Notice how the stretching affects your body and your mood.

Creating a Personalized Toolkit

These are just a few examples of the many somatic tools available to help you navigate anxiety and panic. The key is to experiment and find the practices that work best for you. Create a personalized toolkit of go-to exercises that you can easily access when you're feeling overwhelmed.

Don't forget that recovering from trauma is a process rather than a destination. Along the route, obstacles and setbacks are inevitable. But by cultivating a toolbox of somatic skills, you can empower yourself to navigate these challenges with greater ease and resilience, ultimately creating a life that feels more balanced, peaceful, and fulfilling

From Fatigue to Vitality: Practices for Depression and Burnout

The weight of trauma can manifest in our bodies as a persistent fatigue, a heaviness that saps our energy and dims our zest for life. For some, this fatigue can escalate into depression, a debilitating state of emotional numbness and physical exhaustion. Burnout, too, can leave us feeling drained and disconnected, a consequence of chronic stress and overexertion.

Yet, even amidst the darkness of these challenges, your body holds the potential for renewal and revitalization. By incorporating somatic practices into your daily routine, you can gradually awaken your body's innate vitality, nurture your energy reserves, and reclaim a sense of joy and purpose.

Understanding the Mind-Body Connection in Fatigue and Depression

Fatigue and depression are not solely psychological phenomena; they are deeply intertwined with our physiological state. Trauma can dysregulate the nervous system, leading to an imbalance of stress hormones, neurotransmitters, and inflammatory markers. This dysregulation can manifest as a persistent sense of fatigue, low mood, difficulty concentrating, and a lack of motivation.

Somatic practices offer a way to address these imbalances at their root, working with the body's innate intelligence to restore equilibrium and promote healing. By engaging in mindful movement, breathwork, and relaxation techniques, you can re-regulate your nervous system, boost energy levels, and enhance overall well-being.

Somatic Practices for Revitalization

Here are some somatic practices specifically designed to combat fatigue, depression, and burnout:

1. **Energizing Breathwork:**

   - **Breath of Fire (Kapalabhati):** Take a comfortable seat and maintain a straight spine. Breathe in deeply through your nose until all of your lungs are filled. Using your nose to firmly exhale, tense your abdominal muscles.
   - **Breath of Joy (Bhastrika):** Sit comfortably with your spine straight. Inhale deeply through your nose, filling your lungs completely. Exhale forcefully through your nose, contracting your abdominal muscles. Repeat for 1-3 minutes. This invigorating practice can help to clear the respiratory system, boost energy, and uplift mood.

2. **Invigorating Movement:**

   - **Sun Salutations:** This flowing sequence of yoga poses is designed to awaken the body and mind. It combines gentle stretches with dynamic movements, promoting circulation, flexibility, and energy flow.
   - **Tai Chi or Qigong:** These ancient Chinese practices involve slow, graceful movements that are coordinated with the breath. They can help to reduce stress, improve balance and coordination, and cultivate a sense of inner peace.

- **Dancing:** Put on your favorite upbeat music and let your body move freely. Dancing is a joyful way to express yourself, release tension, and boost your mood.

3. **Restorative Yoga:**

- **Legs-Up-the-Wall Pose:** Lie on your back with your buttocks against a wall and your legs extended up the wall. This pose can help to reduce fatigue, improve circulation, and calm the nervous system.
- **Supported Child's Pose:** Kneel on the floor and bring your big toes together. Sit back on your heels and fold forward, resting your forehead on a block or pillow. This gentle pose can help to soothe the nervous system and promote relaxation.

4. **Grounding Practices:**

- **Barefoot Walking:** Walk barefoot on grass, sand, or earth to connect with the grounding energy of the Earth. This practice can help to reduce stress, improve sleep, and enhance overall well-being.
- **Mindful Nature Connection:** Spend time in nature, observing the sights, sounds, and smells around you. This can help to reduce rumination, promote relaxation, and foster a sense of connection to something larger than yourself.

Beyond the Mat: Lifestyle Changes for Sustained Vitality

In addition to these somatic practices, making certain lifestyle changes can also contribute to increased energy and improved mood:

- **Nutrition:** Eat a balanced diet rich in whole foods, fruits, vegetables, and lean protein. Avoid processed foods, sugar, and excessive caffeine, which can contribute to energy crashes and mood swings.
- **Sleep Hygiene:** Establish a consistent sleep schedule, create a relaxing bedtime routine, and ensure your bedroom is dark, quiet, and cool.
- **Stress Management:** Identify and resolve the sources of stress in your life to practise stress management. This could entail establishing limits, assigning responsibilities, or asking a therapist or counselor for assistance.

- **Social Connection:** Connect with loved ones, join a support group, or engage in activities that bring you joy and a sense of community. Social connection is essential for mental health and well-being.

Understand that the transition from exhaustion to vitality is a slow one. Have patience with yourself and acknowledge your little accomplishments as you go. Your body, mind, and spirit can be nourished by implementing these somatic practices and lifestyle modifications into your daily routine, which will open the door to a more vibrant and satisfying life.

CHAPTER 7

INTEGRATING SOMATICS INTO YOUR LIFE: BEYOND THE EXERCISES

As you've progressed through the pages of this book, you've encountered a diverse array of somatic exercises designed to release tension, soothe your nervous system, and foster a deeper connection with your body. These practices, while potent in their own right, are not meant to be isolated events. True healing comes from integrating somatic principles into the fabric of your daily life, weaving them into the routines, habits, and choices that shape your existence.

Creating a Sustainable Somatic Practice

The beauty of somatic exercises lies in their accessibility and flexibility. Unlike rigid fitness regimes, they can be seamlessly woven into your existing routines. This chapter is your guide to creating a sustainable somatic practice that nurtures your well-being without adding extra stress or pressure to your life.

1. **Start Small and Build Gradually:** Don't feel obligated to cram multiple exercises into your day. Begin with a few minutes of mindful breathing or a gentle stretch when you wake up or before bed. As you get more used to it, progressively extend the time or frequency of your practice.

2. **Embrace Flexibility:** Life is unpredictable, and there will be days when sticking to a strict schedule is simply not possible. Instead of viewing this as a failure, embrace the flexibility of somatic practices. Don't be hard on yourself if you skip a day. Just pick up the next day where you left off.

3. **Listen to Your Body:** Your body is your wisest guide. Pay attention to its signals and adjust your practice accordingly. Some days you may crave vigorous movement, while other days, gentle stretching or restorative yoga may be more appropriate. Honor your body's needs, and don't push yourself beyond your limits.

4. **Make it Enjoyable:** The more you enjoy your somatic practice, the more likely you are to stick with it. Experiment with different exercises and find what resonates with you. Maybe you love dancing to your favorite music, or perhaps you find solace in a quiet meditation. The key is to make it a pleasurable experience, not a chore.

Somatic Mindfulness in Everyday Life

Somatic practices are not confined to the yoga mat or meditation cushion. They can be seamlessly integrated into your daily activities, enhancing your awareness and well-being in every moment.

1. **Mindful Walking:** As you walk, pay attention to the sensations in your feet as they make contact with the ground. Feel the roll of your foot from heel to toe, and the gentle swing of your arms. Take note of the sights, sounds, and rhythm of your breathing.
2. **Mindful Eating:** Slow down and savor each bite, paying attention to the flavors, textures, and aromas of your food. When you're comfortably full, stop eating and pay attention to how your body feels.
3. **Mindful Working:** Take short breaks throughout your workday to check in with your body and breath. Stand up and stretch, take a few deep breaths, or simply close your eyes and focus on the sensations in your body. This can help to reduce stress, improve focus, and enhance productivity.

Embracing a Trauma-Informed Lifestyle

A trauma-informed lifestyle goes beyond individual somatic practices. It involves creating a supportive environment for your healing journey, both internally and externally.

1. **Prioritize Self-Care:** Make self-care a priority by scheduling time for activities that uplift your body, mind, and soul. This might include spending time in nature, listening to music, taking a warm bath, or connecting with loved ones.
2. **Set Healthy Boundaries:** Learn to say no to things that drain your energy or don't align with your values. Communicate your needs clearly and assertively, and create space for solitude and self-reflection.
3. **Seek Assistance:** Never hesitate to ask for assistance when you need it. Connect with a therapist, support group, or trusted friend who can offer guidance, encouragement, and a listening ear.

Your Ongoing Healing Journey

Integrating somatic practices into your life is an ongoing journey of self-discovery and healing. It's about embracing your body as a source of wisdom and resilience, and cultivating a deeper connection to your inner landscape.

Remember, there is no right or wrong way to practice somatics. The most important thing is to find practices that resonate with you and that you can incorporate into your daily life in a sustainable way. Be kind and patient with yourself as you proceed on this journey. Celebrate your successes, learn from your challenges, and trust that your body is always guiding you towards greater healing and wholeness.

Creating A Sustainable Practice: Tips For Consistency And Ease

Consistency is key to reaping the full benefits of somatic practices for trauma recovery. However, establishing a sustainable routine can be challenging, especially when juggling the demands of daily life and the emotional intensity of healing. This chapter offers practical tips and strategies to help you weave somatic exercises seamlessly into your routine, fostering a sense of ease and consistency that empowers your journey towards well-being.

1. **Start Small and Build Gradually:**

The adage "slow and steady wins the race" holds particularly true for establishing a new habit. Instead of overwhelming yourself with an ambitious schedule, begin with small, manageable steps. Set aside 5-10 minutes each day for a single somatic exercise that resonates with you. As you get more accustomed to it, progressively extend the time or frequency of your practice.

2. **Anchor Your Practice:**

Linking your somatic exercises to existing habits can make them easier to remember and incorporate. For example, you might practice deep breathing exercises while you brush your teeth in the morning, or do a quick body scan before bed. By anchoring your practice to existing routines, you're more likely to make it a consistent part of your day.

3. **Embrace Flexibility:**

Life is full of unexpected twists and turns, and there will be days when you simply can't stick to your planned routine. Instead of viewing this as a failure, embrace the flexibility of somatic practices. If you miss a day, Don't be hard on yourself if you skip a day. Just pick up the next day where you left off. Remember, consistency doesn't mean perfection; it means showing up for yourself as often as you can.

4. Prioritize Pleasure:

Somatic practices should be enjoyable, not a chore. If you dread your practice, it's unlikely to become a sustainable habit. Experiment with different exercises and techniques until you find those that bring you joy and a sense of ease. Whether it's dancing to your favorite music, taking a mindful walk in nature, or indulging in a soothing bath, prioritize activities that nourish your body and soul.

5. Create a Sacred Space:

Designate a specific area in your home where you can practice your somatic exercises. This could be a quiet corner of your bedroom, a cozy nook in your living room, or even a designated chair. Fill this space with items that bring you comfort and joy, such as candles, soft blankets, or inspiring artwork. By creating a sacred space for your practice, you'll cultivate a sense of ritual and intention, making it easier to prioritize your well-being.

6. Track Your Progress:

Keep a journal or use a habit tracker to monitor your practice. Note how you feel before, during, and after each exercise. Tracking your progress can help you identify patterns, celebrate your successes, and stay motivated on your journey.

7. Be Kind to Yourself:

Self-compassion is essential for a sustainable somatic practice. Don't judge yourself for missing a day or struggling with a particular exercise. Understand that recovery is a journey, not a destination. Show yourself the same consideration and compassion that you would show a close friend.

8. Seek Support:

Connecting with others who are also practicing somatic exercises can be a powerful source of support and encouragement. Consider joining a group class, finding a practice partner, or seeking guidance from a somatic therapist. Sharing your experiences and challenges with others can help you stay motivated and accountable.

9. **Celebrate Your Successes:**

Take time to acknowledge and celebrate your progress, no matter how small it may seem. Recognize the effort you're putting into your healing journey, and be proud of yourself for taking steps to prioritize your well-being.

Beyond the 10-Minute Mark: Integrating Somatics into Daily Life

Remember, somatic practices are not limited to the dedicated time you set aside for your formal practice. You can integrate somatic awareness into everyday activities, infusing your life with mindfulness and presence.

- **Mindful Showering:** Pay attention to the sensations of the water on your skin, the scent of the soap, and the sound of the water running. Notice how your body feels as you wash away the day's stress and tension.
- **Mindful Eating:** Enjoy every bite of your food by taking time to appreciate its flavours, textures, and aromas. As you eat, pay attention to how your body feels, and stop when you're satisfied but not overstuffed.
- **Mindful Walking:** As you walk, pay attention to the sensations in your feet as they make contact with the ground. Notice the rhythm of your breath and the gentle swaying of your arms.
- **Mindful Working:** Take short breaks throughout your workday to check in with your body and breath. Stand up and stretch, take a few deep breaths, or simply close your eyes and focus on the sensations in your body.

By weaving somatic awareness into the fabric of your daily life, you'll cultivate a deeper connection to your body and its wisdom. You'll learn to recognize and respond to your needs more effectively, creating a foundation for lasting resilience and well-being.

Somatic Mindfulness In Daily Life: Integrating Presence Into Your Routine

The true power of somatic practices lies not in isolated exercises but in their seamless integration into the fabric of our daily lives. By weaving mindful embodiment into our routines, we can cultivate a deeper sense of presence, reduce stress, and enhance our overall well-being. This chapter offers practical guidance on how to infuse somatic mindfulness into everyday activities, transforming mundane moments into opportunities for healing and connection.

1. **Mindful Waking:**

Start your day by tuning into your body. Before even getting out of bed, take a few moments to notice the sensations in your body. Feel the weight of your body against the mattress, the rise and fall of your chest as you breathe, the gentle pulsing of your heart.

- Practical Step: As you begin to move, do so slowly and deliberately. Avoid rushing into the day. Instead, take a few minutes to stretch, yawn, or simply sit at the edge of your bed and breathe deeply.

2. **Mindful Showering or Bathing:**

Transform your daily cleansing ritual into a mindful experience. Notice the temperature of the water on your skin, the scent of the soap, and the sound of the water running. Pay attention to the feeling of your hands moving over your body, massaging the soap into your skin and rinsing it away.

- Practical Step: As you wash, focus on the present moment. Avoid thinking about your to-do list or replaying events from yesterday. Simply be with the sensations of your body in the shower or bath.

3. **Mindful Eating:**

Eating can be a deeply grounding and nourishing experience when approached with mindfulness. Before you take your first bite, pause and appreciate the appearance of your food. Notice its colors, textures, and aromas. As you eat, slow down and savor each bite, paying attention to the flavors and sensations in your mouth.

- Practical Step: In between bites, set down your fork or spoon and take a deep breath. As you consume, take note of how your body feels. Do you feel satisfied right now? Feeling hungry? Complete?

4. **Mindful Walking:**

Walking is a simple yet powerful way to integrate mindfulness into your day. As you walk, pay attention to the sensations in your feet as they make contact with the ground. Feel the heel strike, the roll of your foot, and the push-off of your toes. Notice the rhythm of your breath and the gentle swaying of your arms.

- Practical Step: If you find your mind wandering, gently bring it back to the sensations of walking. You can also try counting your steps or repeating a mantra as you walk.

5. **Mindful Working:**

Even in the midst of a busy workday, you can incorporate somatic mindfulness. Take short breaks to stretch, breathe deeply, or simply close your eyes and tune into your body.

- Practical Step: Set a timer to remind yourself to take breaks throughout the day. Use these breaks to check in with your body, noticing any areas of tension or discomfort. If you find yourself feeling overwhelmed, take a few minutes to practice a grounding exercise or breathwork technique.

6. **Mindful Communication:**

Somatic mindfulness can also enhance your interactions with others. When you're engaged in conversation, pay attention to your body language and tone of voice. Notice how your body feels in response to what the other person is saying.

- Practical Step: Practice active listening, giving the other person your full attention. Notice any sensations or emotions that arise within you as you listen. Respond with authenticity and compassion, honoring both your own needs and the needs of the other person.

7. **Mindful Relaxation:**

At the end of the day, take some time to unwind and relax. This might involve taking a warm bath, reading a book, listening to calming music, or spending time in nature.

- Practical Step: As you relax, pay attention to the sensations in your body. Notice how your muscles soften, your breath deepens, and your mind quiets. Give yourself permission to let go completely and give in to the here and now.

Building a Sustainable Practice

Integrating somatic mindfulness into your daily life is an ongoing process. It requires patience, commitment, and a willingness to experiment with different practices. Be kind to yourself as you explore what works best for you, and remember that even small moments of mindfulness can have a profound impact on your well-being. As you continue to practice, you'll discover that somatic mindfulness is not just a set of exercises but a way of being in the world. It's about cultivating a deeper connection to your body, your emotions, and the present moment. By embracing somatic mindfulness, you can transform your relationship with yourself and the world around you, creating a life that feels more vibrant, meaningful, and fulfilling.

Embracing a Trauma-Informed Lifestyle: Prioritizing Self-Care and Healing

The path to recovery from trauma extends far beyond isolated exercises or therapy sessions. It involves a fundamental shift in how we approach our lives, a conscious choice to prioritize self-care, cultivate supportive relationships, and create a safe and nurturing environment for healing. Embracing a trauma-informed lifestyle is not a quick fix but a lifelong commitment to honoring your body, mind, and spirit.

What is a Trauma-Informed Lifestyle?

A trauma-informed lifestyle is rooted in an understanding of how trauma affects the nervous system and the body as a whole. It acknowledges that past experiences can shape our perceptions, behaviors, and relationships in profound ways. By embracing a trauma-informed lens, we can learn to recognize our triggers, respond to stress in healthy ways, and create a life that feels safe, empowered, and fulfilling.

This approach extends beyond individual actions to encompass our relationships, work environments, and communities. It recognizes that healing is not just an individual endeavor but a collective responsibility. By fostering trauma-informed environments, we can create a world that supports and empowers survivors on their healing journeys.

Practical Steps for Embracing a Trauma-Informed Lifestyle

1. **Prioritize Self-Care:**

Self-care is not a luxury; it's a necessity, especially for those healing from trauma. Schedule time each day for mental, physical, and spiritual growth. This might include:

- **Movement:** Engage in gentle movement practices like yoga, tai chi, or qigong.
- **Rest:** Prioritize getting enough sleep and allow yourself to rest when you're feeling tired.
- **Nutrition:** Nourish your body with whole, unprocessed foods that support your energy and well-being.
- **Connection:** Spend time with loved ones who make you feel safe and supported.
- **Creativity:** Engage in creative activities like painting, writing, or music.
- **Mindfulness:** Practice mindfulness meditation or other techniques to cultivate present moment awareness.
- **Nature:** Spend time in nature, connecting with the beauty and tranquillity of the natural world.

2. **Set Healthy Boundaries:**

It might be challenging to establish and sustain healthy boundaries after trauma. However, boundaries are essential for protecting your energy, preventing overwhelm, and fostering healthy relationships.

- **Learn to say no:** It's okay to decline requests or invitations that don't feel right for you.
- **Speak your truth:** Express your needs and feelings honestly and directly.
- **Protect your personal space:** Create physical and emotional space for yourself to recharge and de-stress.
- **Surround yourself with positive people:** Cultivate relationships with people who respect your boundaries and support your well-being.

3. **Seek Support When Needed:**

Healing from trauma is not a solo journey. Don't hesitate to reach out for support from trusted friends, family members, or professionals.

- **Therapy:** A therapist can provide a safe and supportive space to process your experiences and develop coping mechanisms.
- **Support groups:** Connecting with others who have experienced trauma can be incredibly empowering and validating.
- **Community resources:** Explore trauma-informed resources in your community, such as yoga classes, meditation groups, or support groups.

4. Cultivate Safety and Trust:

For trauma rehabilitation to occur, a feeling of safety must be created. This involves not only protecting yourself from physical harm but also creating an emotional environment that feels safe and nurturing.

- **Surround yourself with positive influences:** Embrace a positive environment by surrounding yourself with individuals who encourage and boost your self-esteem.
- **Limit exposure to triggers:** Be mindful of the media you consume, the conversations you engage in, and the environments you spend time in. If something triggers you, give yourself permission to step away and take care of yourself.
- **Practice self-compassion:** Treat yourself with kindness, particularly when you're having troubles. Remember that healing is a process, and there will be ups and downs along the way.

5. Celebrate Your Wins:

Every move you take in the direction of recovery is a triumph to be proud of. Reward yourself for whatever progress you make, no matter how tiny.

Appreciate the bravery required to confront your pain and welcome the healing process. Celebrate your fortitude, tenacity, and steadfast dedication to your wellbeing.

The Journey Continues:

Living a trauma-informed lifestyle means committing to honouring your body, mind, and spirit for the rest of your life. It's about building a life that you feel confident in, secure in, and consistent with your principles. You can create the conditions for long-lasting healing and transformation by putting self-care first, establishing healthy boundaries, getting help, and building a culture of safety and trust.

Recall that you are not travelling alone. Numerous communities and services are at your disposal to assist you. In addition to helping oneself heal, adopting a trauma-informed lifestyle makes the world a more sympathetic and understanding place.

Your Ongoing Journey Of Embodied Healing

As you close the final pages of this book, take a moment to reflect on the profound journey you have embarked upon. You have explored the depths of your inner landscape, learned to listen to your body's wisdom, and cultivated a toolbox of somatic practices to support your healing and growth. But your journey doesn't end here; it is an ongoing process of self-discovery, transformation, and empowerment. Throughout these pages, you have delved into the intricate connection between mind and body, recognizing how trauma can leave its mark on both our emotional and physical well-being. You have learned how the nervous system, the body's command center, can become dysregulated in the aftermath of trauma, leading to a host of physical and emotional symptoms.

But you have also discovered the transformative power of somatic practices to re-regulate the nervous system, release stored tension, and cultivate a deeper connection to your body's innate wisdom. Through grounding techniques, breathwork, mindful movement, and self-compassion, you have begun to reclaim your sense of safety, agency, and well-being.

The Path of Embodied Healing

The journey of healing from trauma is not a linear path; it's a winding road with twists, turns, and unexpected detours. There will be days when you feel strong and empowered, and other days when the weight of the past feels heavy on your shoulders. There will be moments of profound clarity and moments of confusion. There will be setbacks and breakthroughs, moments of joy and moments of sorrow.

But no matter where you are on your journey, remember that healing is a process, not a destination. It takes time, patience, and unwavering self-compassion. Celebrate your accomplishments, no matter how little they might seem. Each step you take towards healing is a victory worth acknowledging.

Embrace the Power of Curiosity

As you continue your journey of embodied healing, approach each new day with a sense of curiosity and openness. Your body is a vast and mysterious landscape, waiting to be explored. Pay attention to its subtle signals, its whispers of wisdom, and its cries for care. Experiment with different somatic practices, discovering what works best for you in each moment.

Keep in mind that there isn't a single fixing strategy that works for everyone. One person's solution might not be another's. Embrace your instincts and go in the direction that feels most natural to you and your requirements.

Building a Supportive Community

Healing from trauma can often feel isolating, but you don't have to walk this path alone. Seek out supportive communities, whether online or in person, where you can connect with others who understand your experiences. Sharing your story, offering support to others, and receiving validation for your feelings can be incredibly empowering.

Consider working with a therapist or other qualified professional who specializes in trauma recovery. They can offer guidance, support, and additional tools to help you navigate the complexities of healing.

Continuing Your Journey of Growth and Transformation

The journey of healing from trauma is not just about recovering from the past; it's also about creating a brighter future. As you continue to practice somatic exercises and embrace a trauma-informed lifestyle, you'll discover new depths of resilience, strength, and inner peace.

You'll learn to recognize your triggers and respond to stress in healthy ways. You'll develop a deeper connection to your body and its wisdom, allowing you to navigate life's challenges with greater ease and confidence. You'll cultivate a sense of self-compassion that allows you to embrace your imperfections and celebrate your strengths.

Ultimately, the journey of embodied healing is about reclaiming your power, your joy, and your innate capacity for love and connection. It's about transforming your relationship with yourself and the world around you, creating a life that feels vibrant, meaningful, and full of possibilities.

Resources for Further Exploration

As you continue your journey of healing and growth, here are some resources that may be helpful:

- **Books:**
    - "The Body Keeps the Score" by Bessel van der Kolk
    - "Waking the Tiger: Healing Trauma" by Peter A. Levine
    - "Trauma and the Body: A Sensorimotor Approach to Psychotherapy" by Pat Ogden
- **Websites:**
    - The National Center for PTSD: https://www.ptsd.va.gov/
    - The Trauma Center at JRI: https://jri.org/
    - The Somatic Experiencing Trauma Institute: https://traumahealing.org/training-event-search/

Remember, you are not alone. There is a vast network of support available to help you on your healing journey. With courage, compassion, and a commitment to self-care, you can overcome the challenges of trauma and create a life that is rich, meaningful, and full of possibilities.

Dear Reader

Thank you so much for selecting this book out of all the options that were presented to you. It means the world to me that you are open to investigating the route of embodied healing. I hope "Quick Somatic Exercises for Trauma Recovery" has given you useful tools and insights to help you on your path to recovery and well-being.

I would appreciate it if you could post a candid review on Amazon in the event that you found this book helpful. Your feedback not only helps other readers discover this resource, but it also helps me to continue creating content that is relevant and meaningful to you

As you continue your journey, remember that healing is a process, not an event. Be patient with yourself, celebrate your progress, and embrace the power of your own body to heal. It would be greatly appreciated if you could recommend this book to someone who is also seeking relief from tension and trauma, please consider sharing this book with them. Together, we can create a ripple effect of healing and empowering the world.

Should you have any questions, comments, or observations about the book, please don't hesitate to reach out to me at speakwithjeromewoodworth@gmail.com value your feedback and am always open to hearing from my readers.

With gratitude,

Jerome Woodworth.

DAILY
FOCUS PLANNER

Date	
Weather	

Morning Checkup

Mood:

Hours Slept:

Hunger level:

Energy level:

Top 3 Tasks

1. _______________________

2. _______________________

3. _______________________

To Do List

Schedule

6 am	
7 am	
8 am	
9 am	
10 am	
11 am	
12 pm	
1 pm	
2 pm	
3 pm	
4 pm	
5 pm	
6 pm	
7 pm	
8 pm	
9 pm	

Meals

Notes

Water

DAILY
FOCUS PLANNER

Date	
Weather	

Morning Checkup

Mood:

Hours Slept:

Hunger level:

Energy level:

Top 3 Tasks

1. _______________________

2. _______________________

3. _______________________

To Do List

Notes

Schedule

6 am	
7 am	
8 am	
9 am	
10 am	
11 am	
12 pm	
1 pm	
2 pm	
3 pm	
4 pm	
5 pm	
6 pm	
7 pm	
8 pm	
9 pm	

Meals

Water

DAILY
FOCUS PLANNER

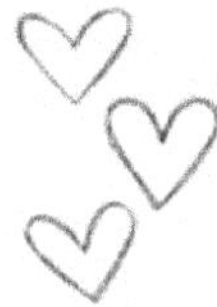

| Date | |
| Weather | |

Morning Checkup

Mood:

Hours Slept:

Hunger level:

Energy level:

Top 3 Tasks

1. ______________________________
2. ______________________________
3. ______________________________

To Do List

- ______________________________ ☐
- ______________________________ ☐
- ______________________________ ☐
- ______________________________ ☐
- ______________________________ ☐
- ______________________________ ☐
- ______________________________ ☐
- ______________________________ ☐
- ______________________________ ☐
- ______________________________ ☐
- ______________________________ ☐
- ______________________________ ☐

Notes

....
....
....
....

Schedule

6 am	
7 am	
8 am	
9 am	
10 am	
11 am	
12 pm	
1 pm	
2 pm	
3 pm	
4 pm	
5 pm	
6 pm	
7 pm	
8 pm	
9 pm	

Meals

Water

DAILY
FOCUS PLANNER

Date	
Weather	

Morning Checkup

Mood:
Hours Slept:
Hunger level:
Energy level:

Top 3 Tasks

1. ___________________________
2. ___________________________
3. ___________________________

To Do List

- ☐
- ☐
- ☐
- ☐
- ☐
- ☐
- ☐
- ☐
- ☐
- ☐
- ☐
- ☐

Notes

....
....
....
....

Schedule

6 am	
7 am	
8 am	
9 am	
10 am	
11 am	
12 pm	
1 pm	
2 pm	
3 pm	
4 pm	
5 pm	
6 pm	
7 pm	
8 pm	
9 pm	

Meals

Water

DAILY
FOCUS PLANNER

Date	
Weather	

Morning Checkup

Mood:

Hours Slept:

Hunger level:

Energy level:

Top 3 Tasks

1. ______________________

2. ______________________

3. ______________________

To Do List

- ☐
- ☐
- ☐
- ☐
- ☐
- ☐
- ☐
- ☐
- ☐
- ☐
- ☐
- ☐

Notes

Schedule

6 am	
7 am	
8 am	
9 am	
10 am	
11 am	
12 pm	
1 pm	
2 pm	
3 pm	
4 pm	
5 pm	
6 pm	
7 pm	
8 pm	
9 pm	

Meals

Water

DAILY
FOCUS PLANNER

Date

Weather

Morning Checkup

Mood:

Hours Slept:

Hunger level:

Energy level:

Top 3 Tasks

1. _______________________________
2. _______________________________
3. _______________________________

To Do List

Notes

Schedule

6 am	
7 am	
8 am	
9 am	
10 am	
11 am	
12 pm	
1 pm	
2 pm	
3 pm	
4 pm	
5 pm	
6 pm	
7 pm	
8 pm	
9 pm	

Meals

Water

DAILY
FOCUS PLANNER

Date

Weather

Morning Checkup

Mood:

Hours Slept:

Hunger level:

Energy level:

Top 3 Tasks

1. _______________________
2. _______________________
3. _______________________

To Do List

- ☐
- ☐
- ☐
- ☐
- ☐
- ☐
- ☐
- ☐
- ☐
- ☐
- ☐

Notes

Schedule

6 am	
7 am	
8 am	
9 am	
10 am	
11 am	
12 pm	
1 pm	
2 pm	
3 pm	
4 pm	
5 pm	
6 pm	
7 pm	
8 pm	
9 pm	

Meals

Water

DAILY
FOCUS PLANNER

Date	
Weather	

Morning Checkup

Mood:

Hours Slept:

Hunger level:

Energy level:

Top 3 Tasks

1. _______________________
2. _______________________
3. _______________________

To Do List

- ☐
- ☐
- ☐
- ☐
- ☐
- ☐
- ☐
- ☐
- ☐
- ☐
- ☐

Notes

Schedule

6 am	
7 am	
8 am	
9 am	
10 am	
11 am	
12 pm	
1 pm	
2 pm	
3 pm	
4 pm	
5 pm	
6 pm	
7 pm	
8 pm	
9 pm	

Meals

Water

DAILY
FOCUS PLANNER

Date	
Weather	

Morning Checkup

Mood:

Hours Slept:

Hunger level:

Energy level:

Top 3 Tasks

1. _______________________

2. _______________________

3. _______________________

To Do List

- ☐
- ☐
- ☐
- ☐
- ☐
- ☐
- ☐
- ☐
- ☐
- ☐
- ☐
- ☐

Notes

. . . .
. . . .
. . . .
. . . .

Schedule

6 am	
7 am	
8 am	
9 am	
10 am	
11 am	
12 pm	
1 pm	
2 pm	
3 pm	
4 pm	
5 pm	
6 pm	
7 pm	
8 pm	
9 pm	

Meals

Water 🥛🥛🥛🥛🥛🥛🥛

DAILY
FOCUS PLANNER

Date	
Weather	

Morning Checkup

Mood:

Hours Slept:

Hunger level:

Energy level:

Top 3 Tasks

1. _______________________
2. _______________________
3. _______________________

To Do List

Notes

Schedule

6 am	
7 am	
8 am	
9 am	
10 am	
11 am	
12 pm	
1 pm	
2 pm	
3 pm	
4 pm	
5 pm	
6 pm	
7 pm	
8 pm	
9 pm	

Meals

Water

DAILY
FOCUS PLANNER

Date	
Weather	

Morning Checkup

Mood:

Hours Slept:

Hunger level:

Energy level:

Top 3 Tasks

1. _______________________

2. _______________________

3. _______________________

To Do List

- [ ] _______________________
- [ ] _______________________
- [ ] _______________________
- [ ] _______________________
- [ ] _______________________
- [ ] _______________________
- [ ] _______________________
- [ ] _______________________
- [ ] _______________________
- [ ] _______________________
- [ ] _______________________

Notes

Schedule

6 am	
7 am	
8 am	
9 am	
10 am	
11 am	
12 pm	
1 pm	
2 pm	
3 pm	
4 pm	
5 pm	
6 pm	
7 pm	
8 pm	
9 pm	

Meals

Water

DAILY
FOCUS PLANNER

Date	
Weather	

Morning Checkup

Mood:

Hours Slept:

Hunger level:

Energy level:

Top 3 Tasks

1. ___________________________
2. ___________________________
3. ___________________________

To Do List

- [ ] _______________________
- [ ] _______________________
- [ ] _______________________
- [ ] _______________________
- [ ] _______________________
- [ ] _______________________
- [ ] _______________________
- [ ] _______________________
- [ ] _______________________
- [ ] _______________________
- [ ] _______________________

Notes

....
....
....
....

Schedule

6 am	
7 am	
8 am	
9 am	
10 am	
11 am	
12 pm	
1 pm	
2 pm	
3 pm	
4 pm	
5 pm	
6 pm	
7 pm	
8 pm	
9 pm	

Meals

Water

DAILY
FOCUS PLANNER

Date	

Weather	

Morning Checkup

Mood:

Hours Slept:

Hunger level:

Energy level:

Top 3 Tasks

1. _______________________
2. _______________________
3. _______________________

To Do List

- ☐
- ☐
- ☐
- ☐
- ☐
- ☐
- ☐
- ☐
- ☐
- ☐
- ☐

Notes

....
....
....
....

Schedule

6 am	
7 am	
8 am	
9 am	
10 am	
11 am	
12 pm	
1 pm	
2 pm	
3 pm	
4 pm	
5 pm	
6 pm	
7 pm	
8 pm	
9 pm	

Meals

Water

DAILY
FOCUS PLANNER

Date	
Weather	

Morning Checkup

Mood:

Hours Slept:

Hunger level:

Energy level:

Top 3 Tasks

1. _______________
2. _______________
3. _______________

To Do List

- [ ] _______________
- [ ] _______________
- [ ] _______________
- [ ] _______________
- [ ] _______________
- [ ] _______________
- [ ] _______________
- [ ] _______________
- [ ] _______________
- [ ] _______________
- [ ] _______________

Notes

Schedule

6 am	
7 am	
8 am	
9 am	
10 am	
11 am	
12 pm	
1 pm	
2 pm	
3 pm	
4 pm	
5 pm	
6 pm	
7 pm	
8 pm	
9 pm	

Meals

Water

DAILY
FOCUS PLANNER

Date	
Weather	

Morning Checkup

Mood:

Hours Slept:

Hunger level:

Energy level:

Top 3 Tasks

1. _______________________

2. _______________________

3. _______________________

To Do List

- ________________ ☐
- ________________ ☐
- ________________ ☐
- ________________ ☐
- ________________ ☐
- ________________ ☐
- ________________ ☐
- ________________ ☐
- ________________ ☐
- ________________ ☐
- ________________ ☐

Notes

....
....
....
....

Schedule

6 am	
7 am	
8 am	
9 am	
10 am	
11 am	
12 pm	
1 pm	
2 pm	
3 pm	
4 pm	
5 pm	
6 pm	
7 pm	
8 pm	
9 pm	

Meals

Water

DAILY
FOCUS PLANNER

Date	
Weather	

Morning Checkup

Mood:

Hours Slept:

Hunger level:

Energy level:

Top 3 Tasks

1. _______________________
2. _______________________
3. _______________________

To Do List

- [ ]
- [ ]
- [ ]
- [ ]
- [ ]
- [ ]
- [ ]
- [ ]
- [ ]
- [ ]
- [ ]

Notes

Schedule

6 am	
7 am	
8 am	
9 am	
10 am	
11 am	
12 pm	
1 pm	
2 pm	
3 pm	
4 pm	
5 pm	
6 pm	
7 pm	
8 pm	
9 pm	

Meals

Water

DAILY
FOCUS PLANNER

Date

Weather

Morning Checkup

Mood:

Hours Slept:

Hunger level:

Energy level:

Top 3 Tasks

1. ______________________
2. ______________________
3. ______________________

To Do List

- [ ] ______________________
- [ ] ______________________
- [ ] ______________________
- [ ] ______________________
- [ ] ______________________
- [ ] ______________________
- [ ] ______________________
- [ ] ______________________
- [ ] ______________________
- [ ] ______________________
- [ ] ______________________
- [ ] ______________________

Notes

Schedule

6 am	
7 am	
8 am	
9 am	
10 am	
11 am	
12 pm	
1 pm	
2 pm	
3 pm	
4 pm	
5 pm	
6 pm	
7 pm	
8 pm	
9 pm	

Meals

Water

DAILY
FOCUS PLANNER

Date	
Weather	

Morning Checkup

Mood:

Hours Slept:

Hunger level:

Energy level:

Top 3 Tasks

1. ___________________________
2. ___________________________
3. ___________________________

To Do List

- ☐
- ☐
- ☐
- ☐
- ☐
- ☐
- ☐
- ☐
- ☐
- ☐
- ☐

Schedule

6 am	
7 am	
8 am	
9 am	
10 am	
11 am	
12 pm	
1 pm	
2 pm	
3 pm	
4 pm	
5 pm	
6 pm	
7 pm	
8 pm	
9 pm	

Meals

Notes

Water

DAILY
FOCUS PLANNER

Date	
Weather	

Morning Checkup

Mood:

Hours Slept:

Hunger level:

Energy level:

Top 3 Tasks

1. _______________________
2. _______________________
3. _______________________

To Do List

- ☐
- ☐
- ☐
- ☐
- ☐
- ☐
- ☐
- ☐
- ☐
- ☐
- ☐
- ☐

Notes

. . . .
. . . .
. . . .
. . . .

Schedule

6 am	
7 am	
8 am	
9 am	
10 am	
11 am	
12 pm	
1 pm	
2 pm	
3 pm	
4 pm	
5 pm	
6 pm	
7 pm	
8 pm	
9 pm	

Meals

Water 🥛 🥛 🥛 🥛 🥛 🥛 🥛

DAILY
FOCUS PLANNER

Date	
Weather	

Morning Checkup

Mood:

Hours Slept:

Hunger level:

Energy level:

Top 3 Tasks

1. ______________________
2. ______________________
3. ______________________

To Do List

- ______________________ ☐
- ______________________ ☐
- ______________________ ☐
- ______________________ ☐
- ______________________ ☐
- ______________________ ☐
- ______________________ ☐
- ______________________ ☐
- ______________________ ☐
- ______________________ ☐
- ______________________ ☐
- ______________________ ☐

Notes

....

....

....

....

Schedule

6 am	
7 am	
8 am	
9 am	
10 am	
11 am	
12 pm	
1 pm	
2 pm	
3 pm	
4 pm	
5 pm	
6 pm	
7 pm	
8 pm	
9 pm	

Meals

Water

DAILY
FOCUS PLANNER

Date	

Weather	

Morning Checkup

Mood:

Hours Slept:

Hunger level:

Energy level:

Top 3 Tasks

1. _______________________
2. _______________________
3. _______________________

To Do List

Notes

Schedule

6 am	
7 am	
8 am	
9 am	
10 am	
11 am	
12 pm	
1 pm	
2 pm	
3 pm	
4 pm	
5 pm	
6 pm	
7 pm	
8 pm	
9 pm	

Meals

Water